I0830704

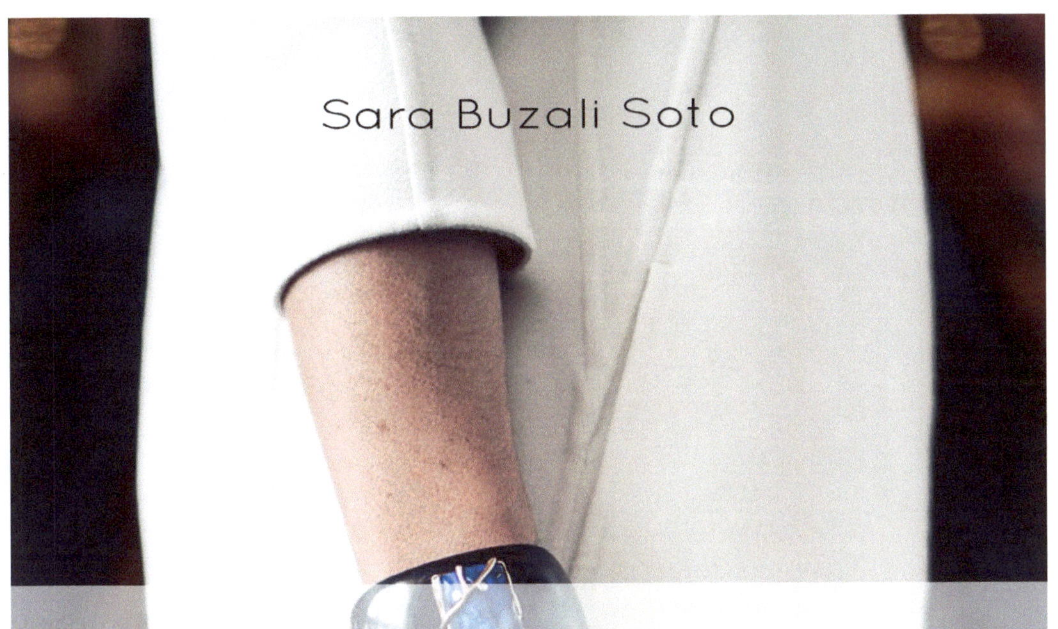

Sara Buzali Soto
Your image
is worth a
thousand words!

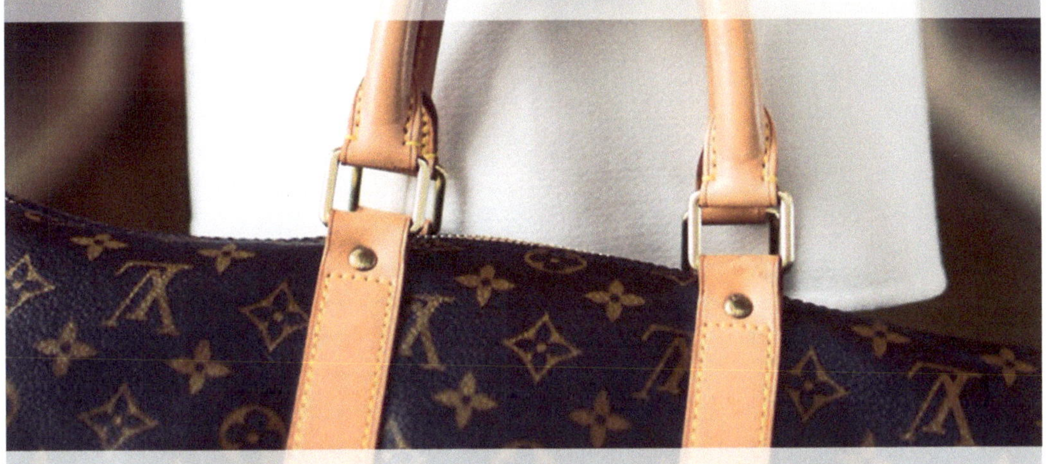

Feel good, live good!

About the author

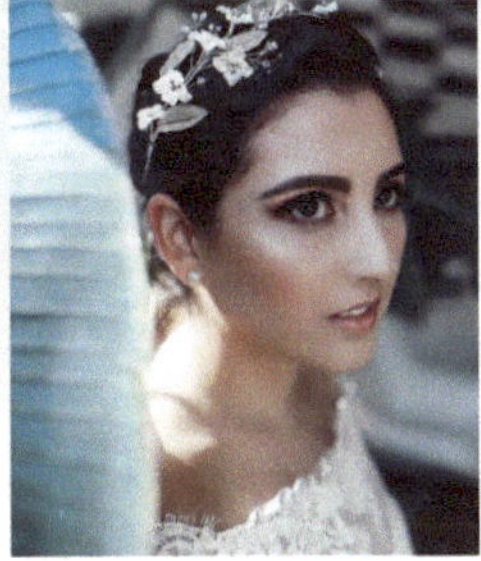

Sara Buzali Soto

She holds a degree in communications by Universidad Panamericana. Master in Public Image with a specialization in Physical Image, and PhD candidate in Public Image by Colegio de Imagen Pública.

Since childhood her interest in acquiring knowledge was remarkable, as well as her concern for society. These are two factors that have led her to continue studying, researching, and writing books. Her topics are related to her profession, but also to philosophical anthropology, and the analysis of today's society.

Her concern for social welfare has made her participate in social service and volunteer projects in South America, Mexico, and the United States.

She has worked in projects with government institutions and the private sector. Through her presence in the digital world, she has revolutionized the image of institutions and people, with her slogan:

"Feel good, live good!"

www.homodeco.com

Acknowledgment

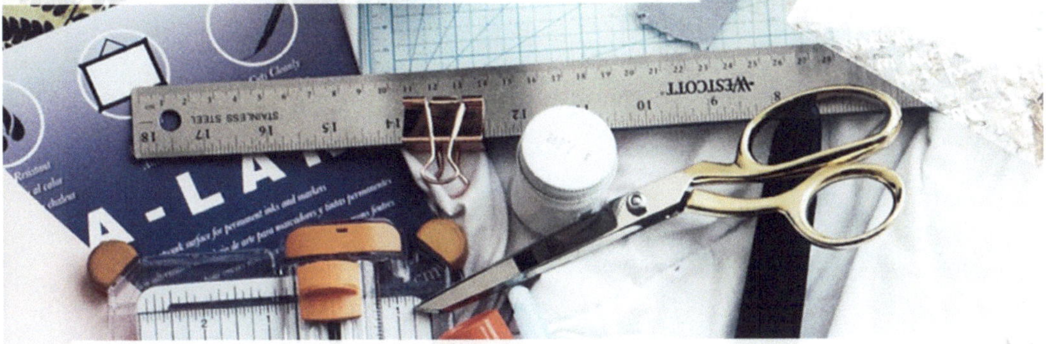

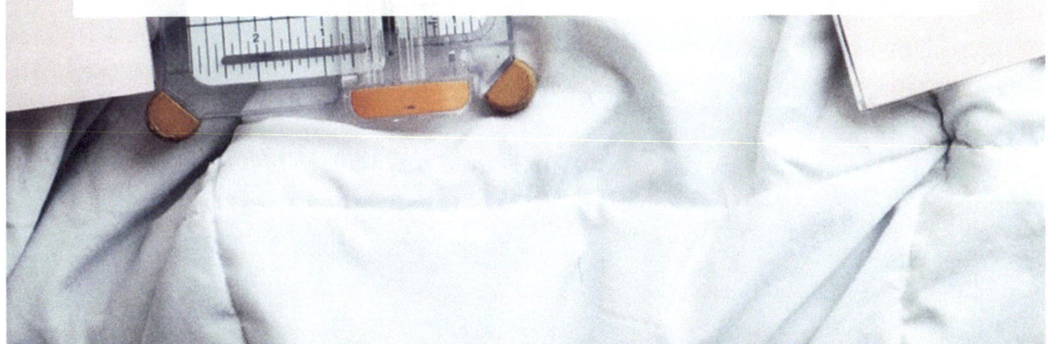

To the first engine for allowing me to be part of this life.

To each member of my family, for always being with me, and believing in my projects.

To my mom, for teaching me how perseverance makes you achieve great things. For supporting me throughout my life, and encouraging me to be a better person.

To my dad, for giving me so much love, for supporting me, and for being by my side in every decision I take.

To my husband Fernando, for inspiring me every day to be a better version of myself.

To my grandmother Elvira, for teaching me how to be closer to God, and for always seeing for my spiritual growth.

To my grandfather Ignacio, for being always by my side and for being an example to follow.

To Bibi, for the immense love he has given to me and for teaching me that whatever you propose, you can achieved.

I especially thank my grandmother Yaya, for instilling in me that passion for communication, for loving others, and for writing.

I love you all!

Index

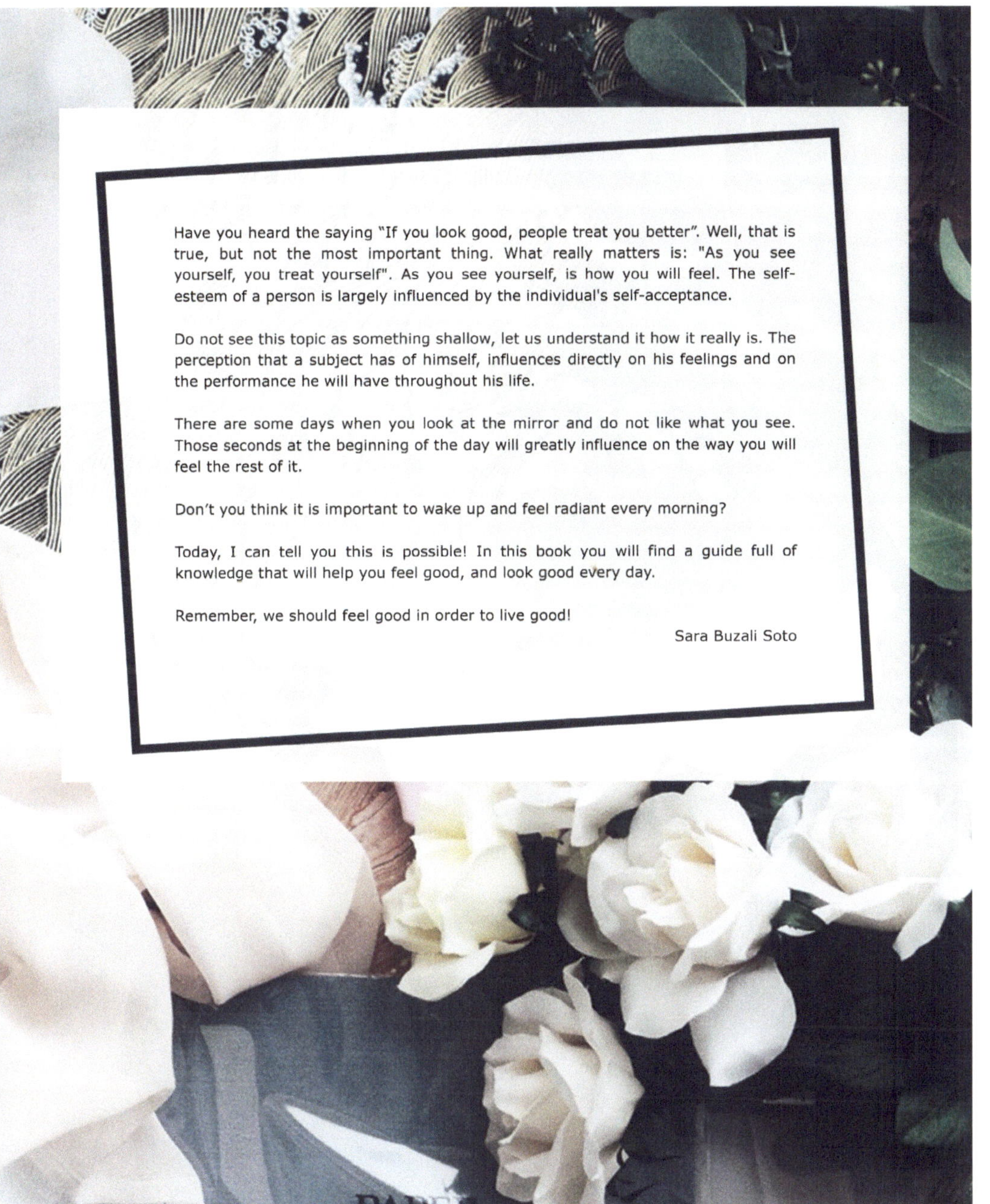

Have you heard the saying "If you look good, people treat you better". Well, that is true, but not the most important thing. What really matters is: "As you see yourself, you treat yourself". As you see yourself, is how you will feel. The self-esteem of a person is largely influenced by the individual's self-acceptance.

Do not see this topic as something shallow, let us understand it how it really is. The perception that a subject has of himself, influences directly on his feelings and on the performance he will have throughout his life.

There are some days when you look at the mirror and do not like what you see. Those seconds at the beginning of the day will greatly influence on the way you will feel the rest of it.

Don't you think it is important to wake up and feel radiant every morning?

Today, I can tell you this is possible! In this book you will find a guide full of knowledge that will help you feel good, and look good every day.

Remember, we should feel good in order to live good!

Sara Buzali Soto

Foreword

First
things
first

This is a practical book so let's go step by step. As step number one, I invite you to take two photos. The first one will be of your face, and the second one of your whole body. It is important that you do not make gestures and that your clothes are tight, that way you are going to be able to see your entire silhouette. This will make work easier. Ready?!

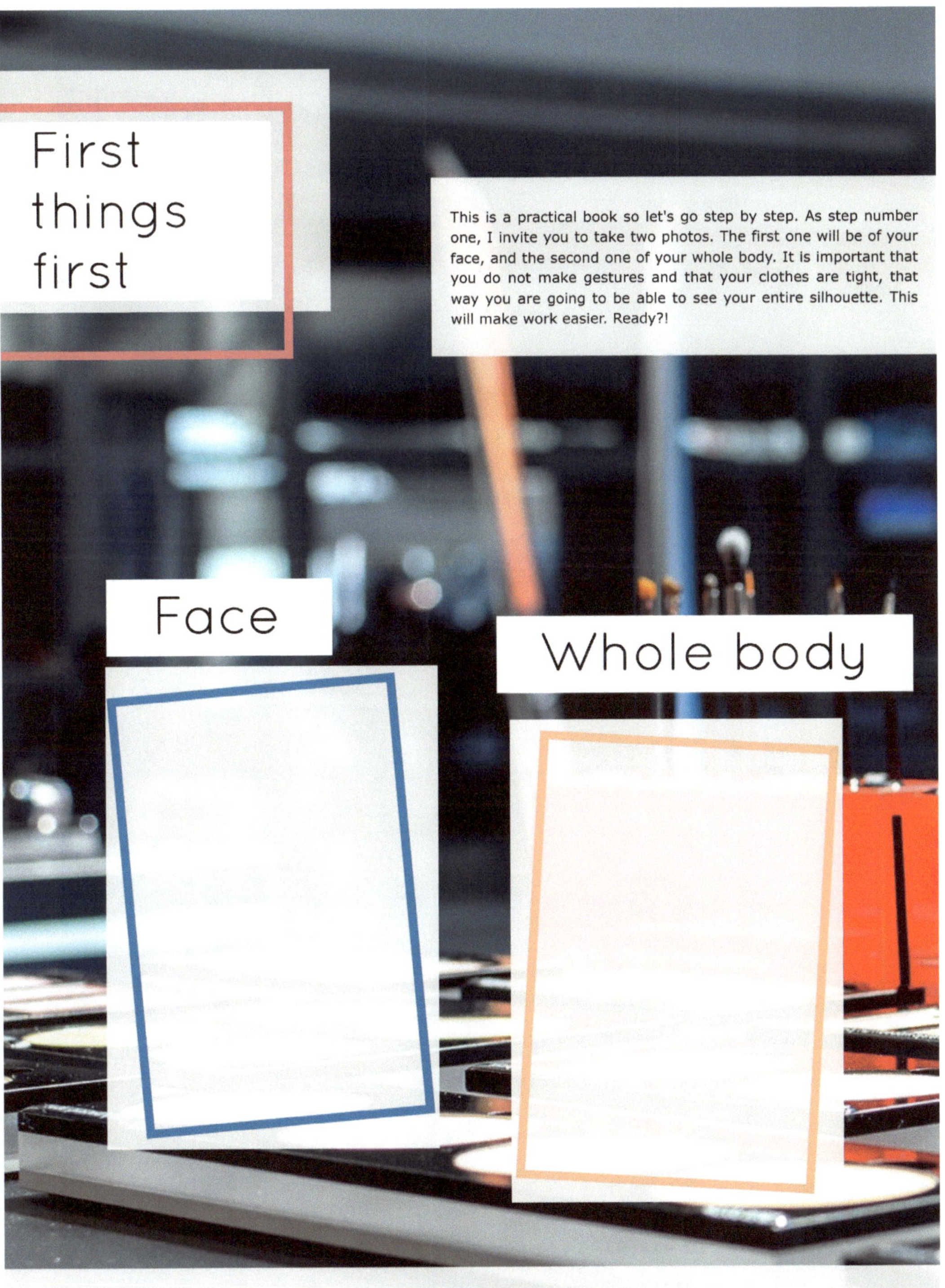

Now, think for a few minutes on how you like to dress. Maybe you are very simple and you prefer comfort, or perhaps you are more crazy and you like to innovate in fashion, or maybe you prefer to look sweeter. The option you choose is perfect, but for the moment just choose one. Later we will talk about styles, and we will discover which one defines you.

If I feel good, I look good

Has it happened to you that when you dress with a special garment, people say: How good you look today!, or How handsome you look! But how about when you wear another outfit and they say: Are you ok?, or Are you feeling bad?

That happened to me, and that is because there is a lot of logic behind. Believe it or not, your image affects directly the perception that others have about you, and as a result affects your self-esteem.

There are colors, silhouettes and shapes that fit some people, but not others. It is for this reason that when you know your colorimetry, your measurements, your shapes, and your style; you will have control over all the stimuli you want to emanate to your audience. Now you will be in charge of what others thinks about you.

I want you to know that this is a long process, which should start from inside the person. This is how we can know its essence, to achieve coherence with what we show to our audience.

My work is not superficial, as some might think, is the opposite. What I do is change people's lives. Together we find all their qualities, so that they can feel good about themselves and as a result: Live good.

An image consultant works with perceptions, with the opinions that others have about something or someone. With what people think about brands, institutions, companies, etc. But do not see it from the outside or as something shallow. There is a lot of work before handling an image. There is an "inside" that must be tapped, so that the "shape" or outside, says what the inside of the product really is. Inside and shape, they work together.

"Your appearance screams what your inside hides." Sara Buzali

The first teacher I had in the field of public image, said that at all times we have to take care of the inside and the outside. This is because if there is a great outside with a cheap inside, the product would lack value. On the other hand, if there is an incredible inside, but with an outside that does not catch the eye, people would never look at the product. That is why inside and outside have the same importance. As a result, there will be coherence and no confusion.

Let us remember the phrase: "Beauty is in the eyes of the beholder." Very true. Although there are several canons of beauty, I want to tell you that for me, beautiful is the person who is kind with their environment. Now, speaking about physical beauty, we all have ours. But sometimes we have to give us a polishing. It is very easy, and that's what this guide and I are for.

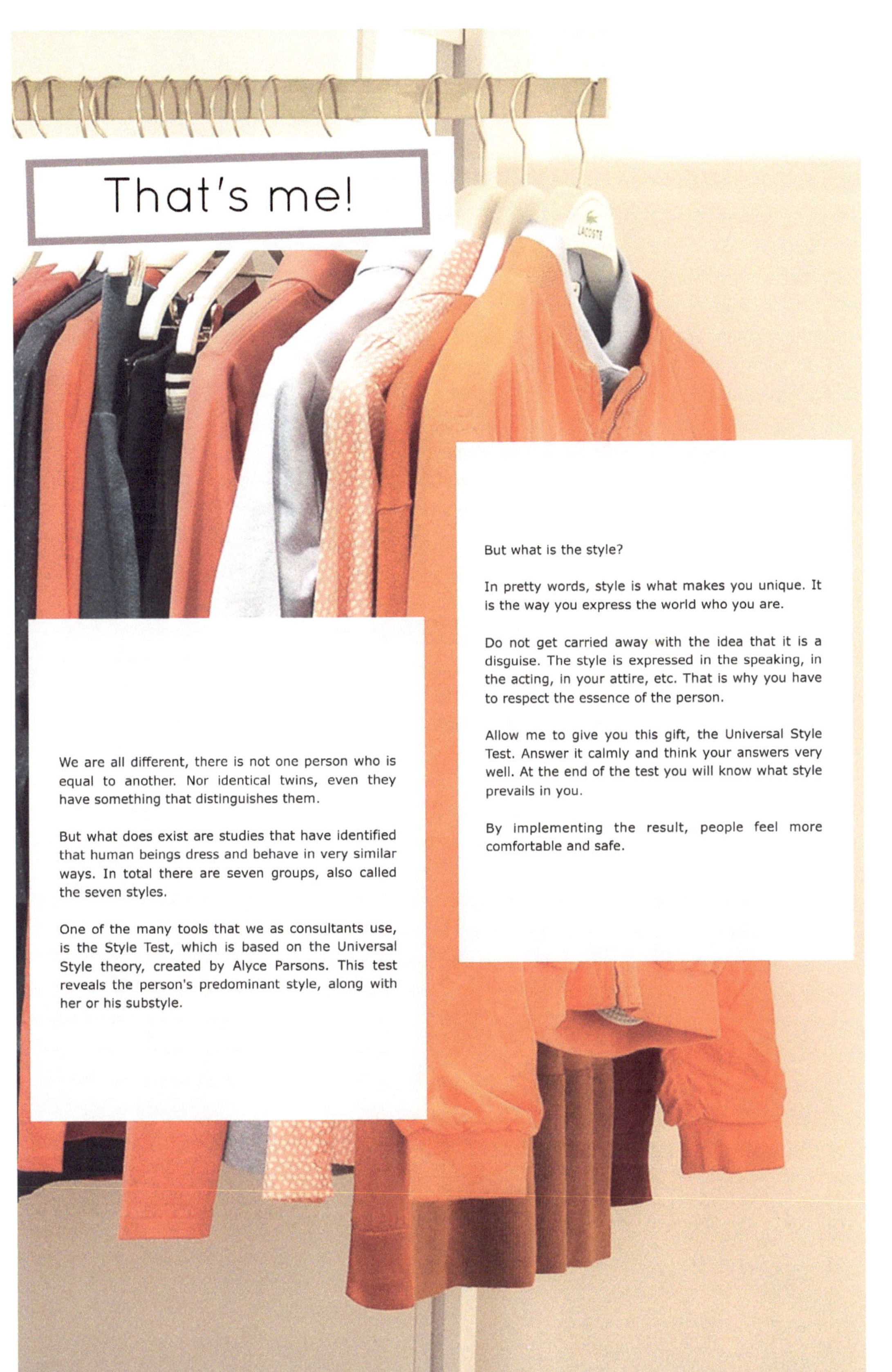

That's me!

We are all different, there is not one person who is equal to another. Nor identical twins, even they have something that distinguishes them.

But what does exist are studies that have identified that human beings dress and behave in very similar ways. In total there are seven groups, also called the seven styles.

One of the many tools that we as consultants use, is the Style Test, which is based on the Universal Style theory, created by Alyce Parsons. This test reveals the person's predominant style, along with her or his substyle.

But what is the style?

In pretty words, style is what makes you unique. It is the way you express the world who you are.

Do not get carried away with the idea that it is a disguise. The style is expressed in the speaking, in the acting, in your attire, etc. That is why you have to respect the essence of the person.

Allow me to give you this gift, the Universal Style Test. Answer it calmly and think your answers very well. At the end of the test you will know what style prevails in you.

By implementing the result, people feel more comfortable and safe.

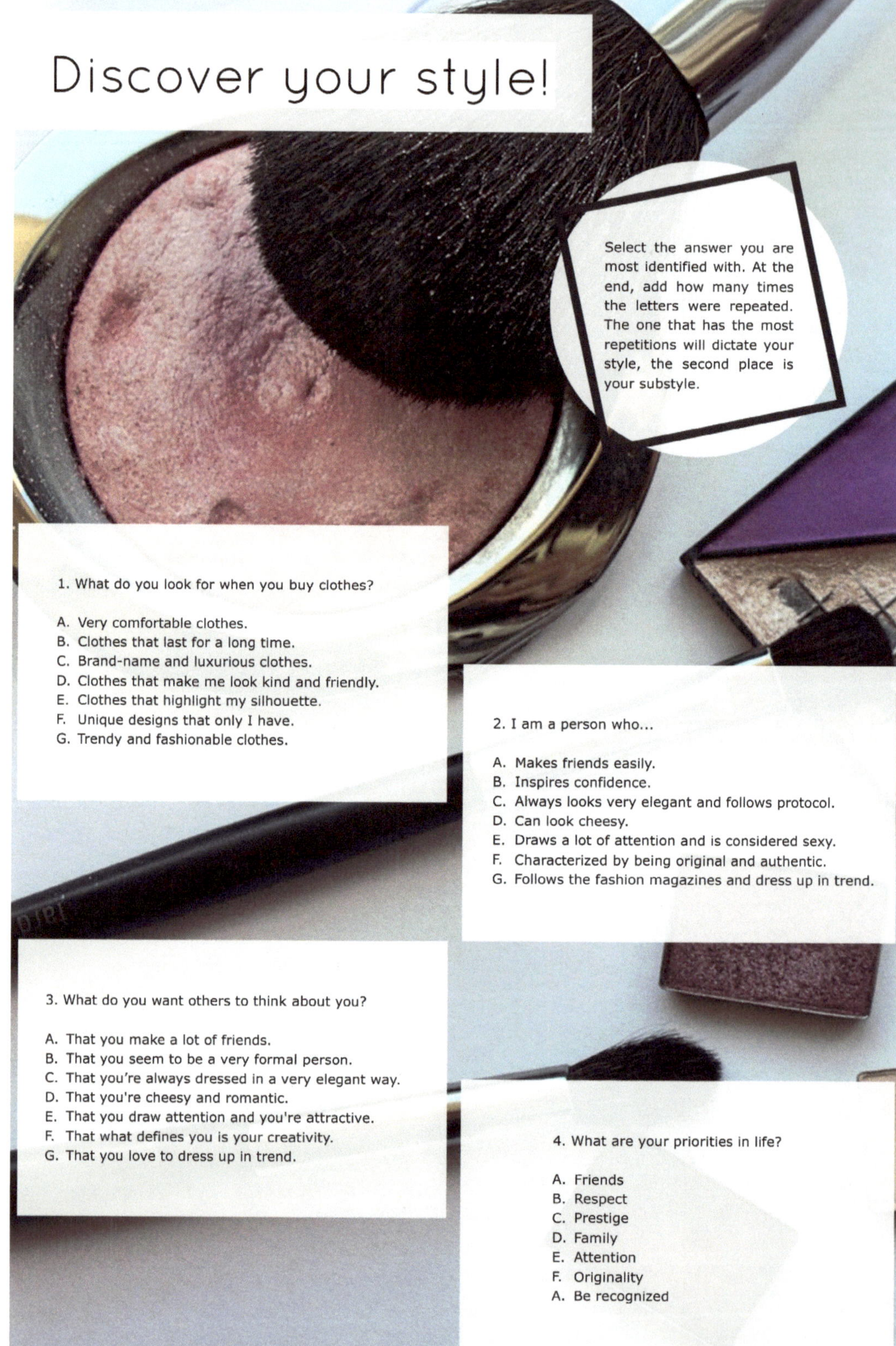

Discover your style!

1. What do you look for when you buy clothes?

A. Very comfortable clothes.
B. Clothes that last for a long time.
C. Brand-name and luxurious clothes.
D. Clothes that make me look kind and friendly.
E. Clothes that highlight my silhouette.
F. Unique designs that only I have.
G. Trendy and fashionable clothes.

2. I am a person who...

A. Makes friends easily.
B. Inspires confidence.
C. Always looks very elegant and follows protocol.
D. Can look cheesy.
E. Draws a lot of attention and is considered sexy.
F. Characterized by being original and authentic.
G. Follows the fashion magazines and dress up in trend.

3. What do you want others to think about you?

A. That you make a lot of friends.
B. That you seem to be a very formal person.
C. That you're always dressed in a very elegant way.
D. That you're cheesy and romantic.
E. That you draw attention and you're attractive.
F. That what defines you is your creativity.
G. That you love to dress up in trend.

4. What are your priorities in life?

A. Friends
B. Respect
C. Prestige
D. Family
E. Attention
F. Originality
A. Be recognized

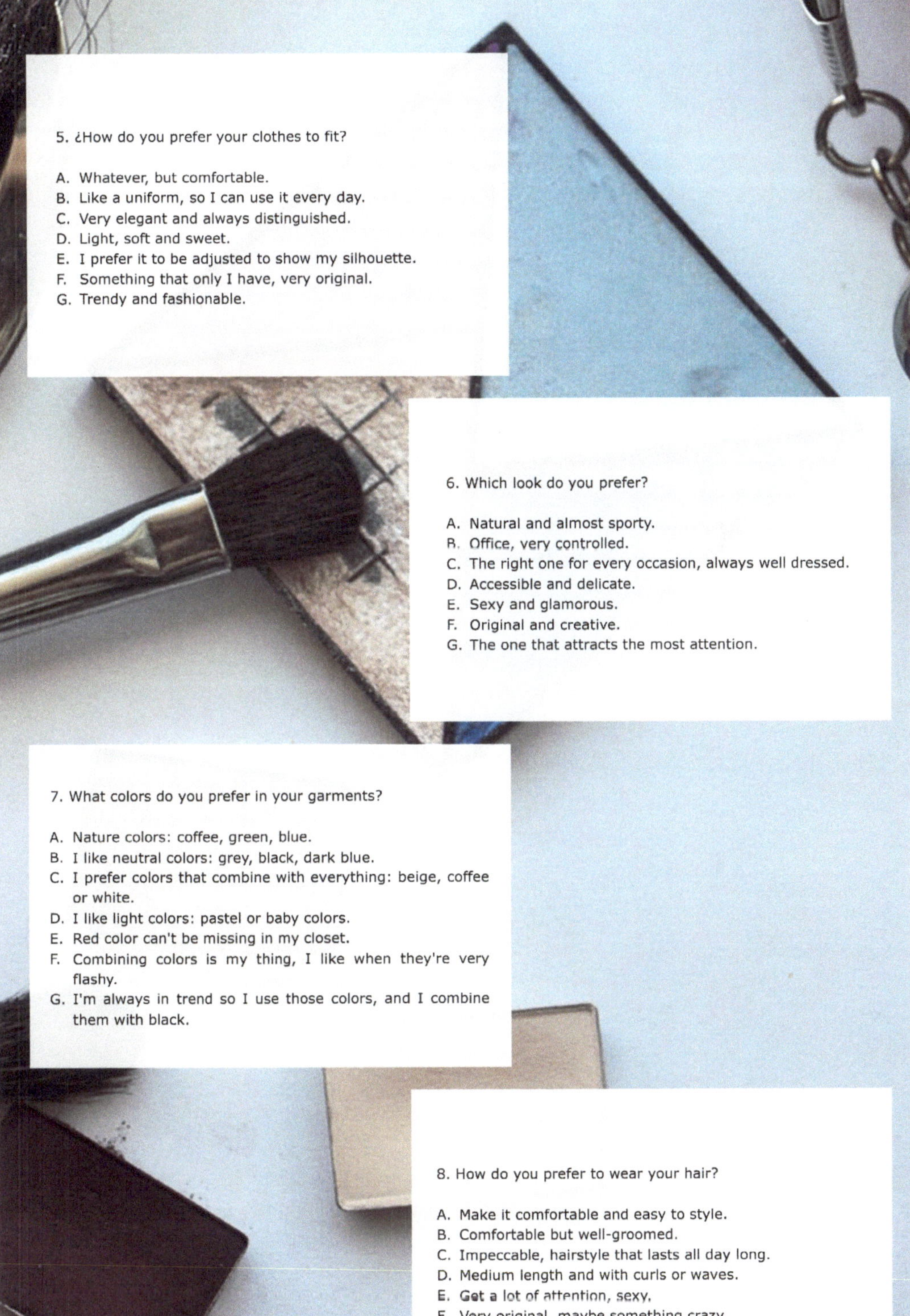

5. ¿How do you prefer your clothes to fit?

A. Whatever, but comfortable.
B. Like a uniform, so I can use it every day.
C. Very elegant and always distinguished.
D. Light, soft and sweet.
E. I prefer it to be adjusted to show my silhouette.
F. Something that only I have, very original.
G. Trendy and fashionable.

6. Which look do you prefer?

A. Natural and almost sporty.
B. Office, very controlled.
C. The right one for every occasion, always well dressed.
D. Accessible and delicate.
E. Sexy and glamorous.
F. Original and creative.
G. The one that attracts the most attention.

7. What colors do you prefer in your garments?

A. Nature colors: coffee, green, blue.
B. I like neutral colors: grey, black, dark blue.
C. I prefer colors that combine with everything: beige, coffee
   or white.
D. I like light colors: pastel or baby colors.
E. Red color can't be missing in my closet.
F. Combining colors is my thing, I like when they're very
   flashy.
G. I'm always in trend so I use those colors, and I combine
   them with black.

8. How do you prefer to wear your hair?

A. Make it comfortable and easy to style.
B. Comfortable but well-groomed.
C. Impeccable, hairstyle that lasts all day long.
D. Medium length and with curls or waves.
E. Get a lot of attention, sexy.
F. Very original, maybe something crazy.
G. Straight-cut and even.

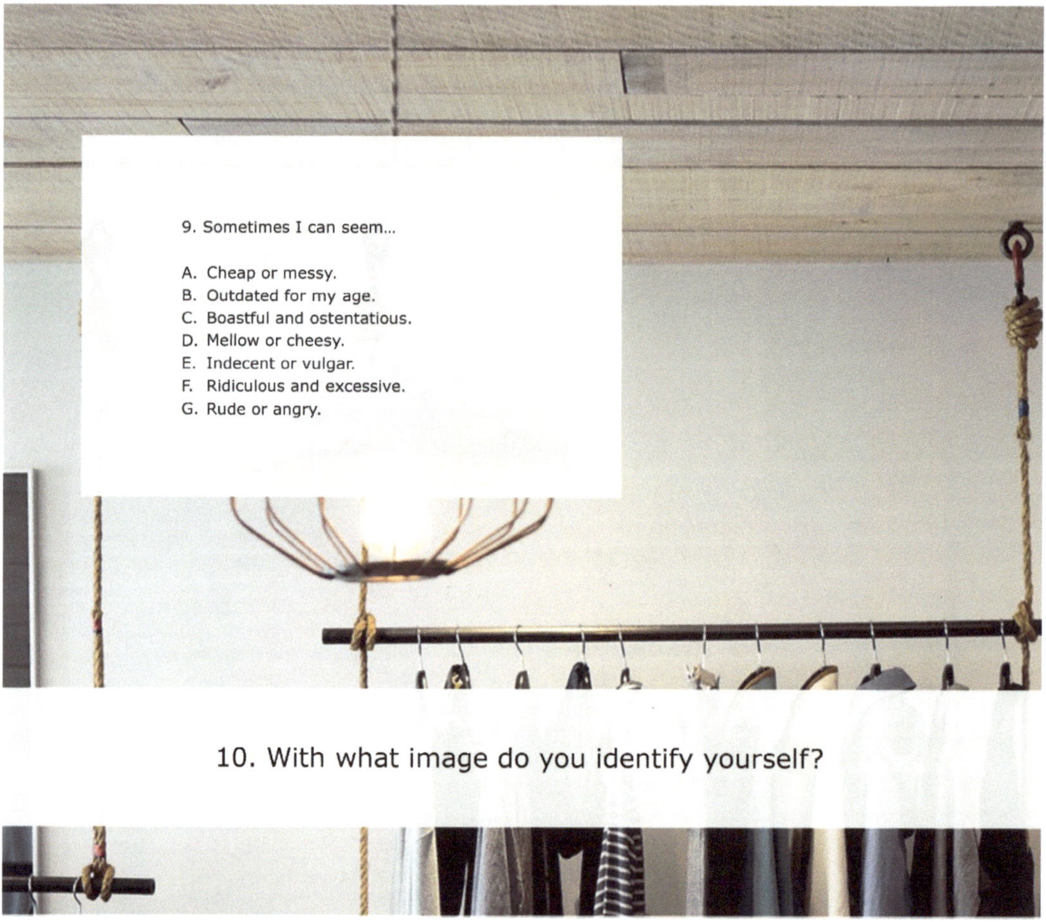

9. Sometimes I can seem...

A. Cheap or messy.
B. Outdated for my age.
C. Boastful and ostentatious.
D. Mellow or cheesy.
E. Indecent or vulgar.
F. Ridiculous and excessive.
G. Rude or angry.

10. With what image do you identify yourself?

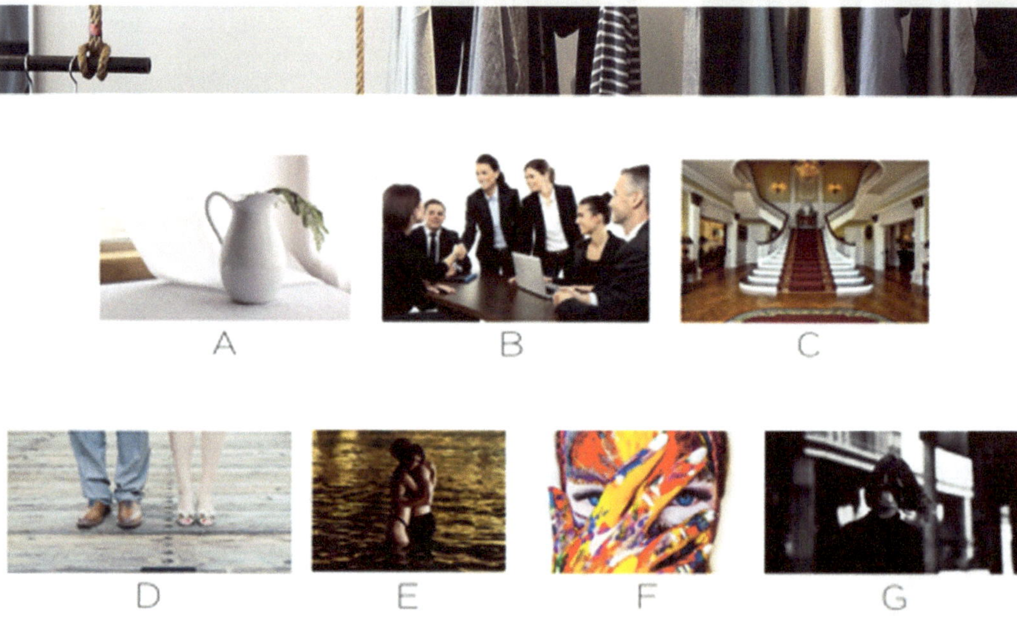

A

B

C

D

E

F

G

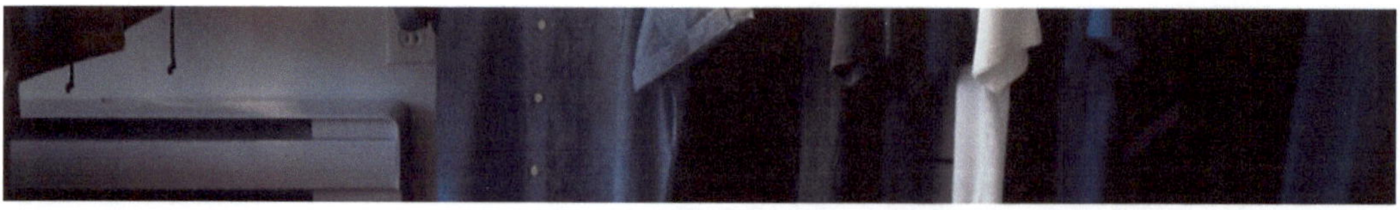

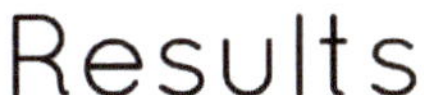

Results

First of all, I want to tell you that this test only reached an approximation of the style that most characterizes you.

However, to know it exactly, you need to go with an image consultant. With deep interviews, quizzes, and more tools, she or he will tell you what style do you belong to.

In addition to orienting yourself with your style and substyle, she or he will help you to implement it and adjust the intensity that goes with your essence.

Results:

• Add the letters that are repeated, the most score will be your style and your substyle.

_______ A. Natural

_______ B. Traditional

_______ C. Elegant

_______ D. Romantic

_______ E. Seductive

_______ F. Creative

_______ G.Dramatic

Now that you know with what style you identify more, we will delve into how they behave and what characterizes them!

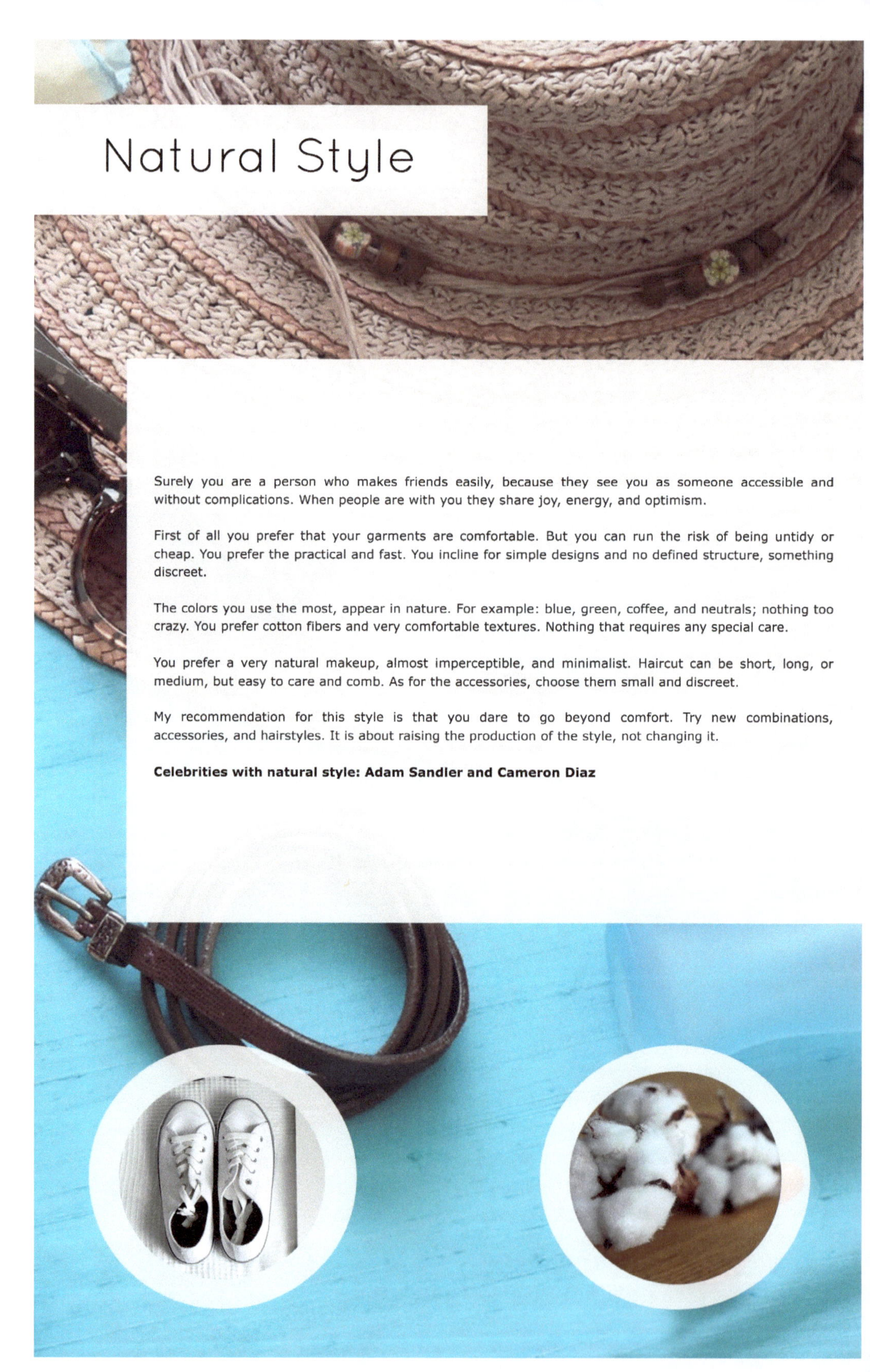

Natural Style

Surely you are a person who makes friends easily, because they see you as someone accessible and without complications. When people are with you they share joy, energy, and optimism.

First of all you prefer that your garments are comfortable. But you can run the risk of being untidy or cheap. You prefer the practical and fast. You incline for simple designs and no defined structure, something discreet.

The colors you use the most, appear in nature. For example: blue, green, coffee, and neutrals; nothing too crazy. You prefer cotton fibers and very comfortable textures. Nothing that requires any special care.

You prefer a very natural makeup, almost imperceptible, and minimalist. Haircut can be short, long, or medium, but easy to care and comb. As for the accessories, choose them small and discreet.

My recommendation for this style is that you dare to go beyond comfort. Try new combinations, accessories, and hairstyles. It is about raising the production of the style, not changing it.

Celebrities with natural style: Adam Sandler and Cameron Diaz

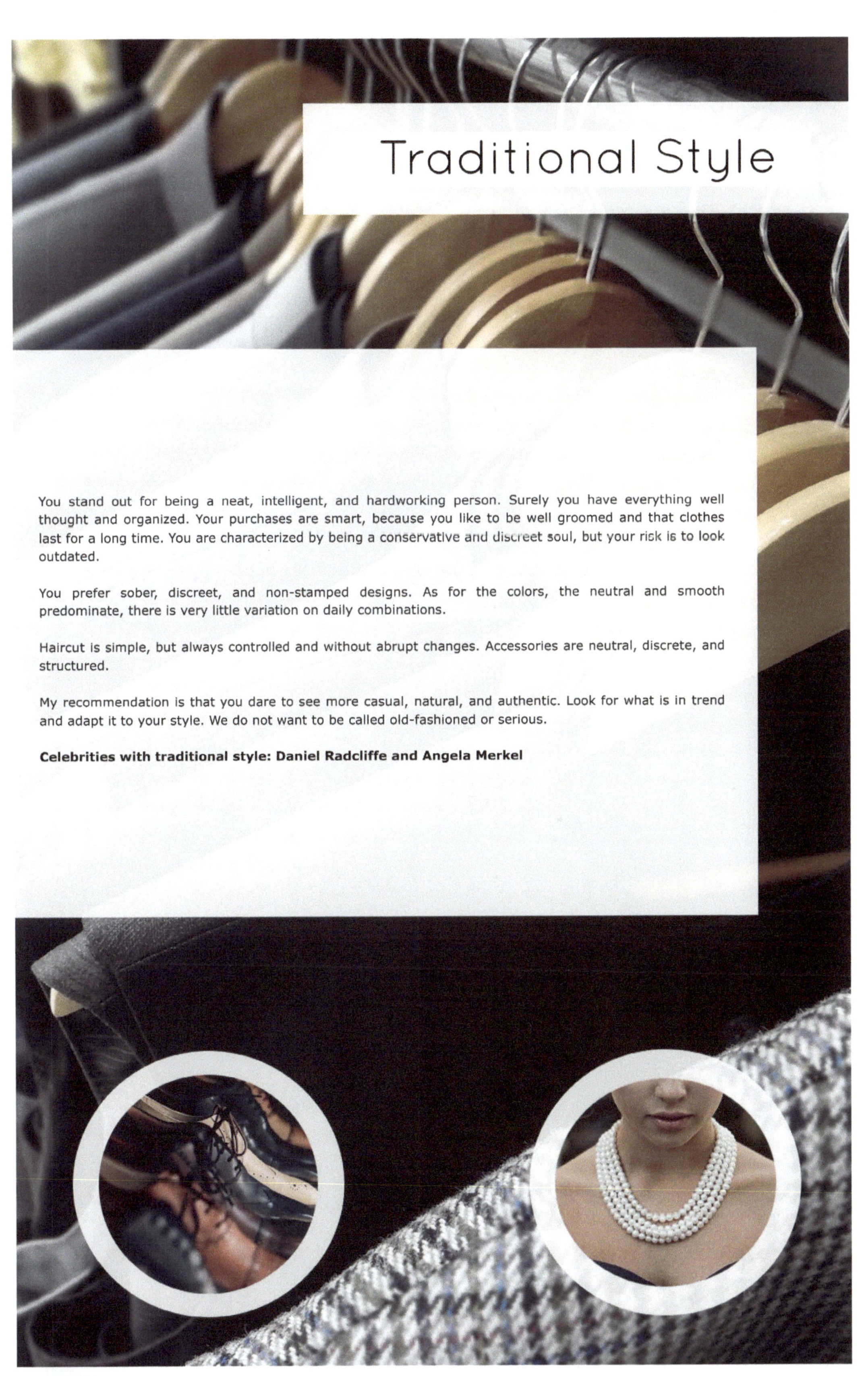

You stand out for being a neat, intelligent, and hardworking person. Surely you have everything well thought and organized. Your purchases are smart, because you like to be well groomed and that clothes last for a long time. You are characterized by being a conservative and discreet soul, but your risk is to look outdated.

You prefer sober, discreet, and non-stamped designs. As for the colors, the neutral and smooth predominate, there is very little variation on daily combinations.

Haircut is simple, but always controlled and without abrupt changes. Accessories are neutral, discrete, and structured.

My recommendation is that you dare to see more casual, natural, and authentic. Look for what is in trend and adapt it to your style. We do not want to be called old-fashioned or serious.

Celebrities with traditional style: Daniel Radcliffe and Angela Merkel

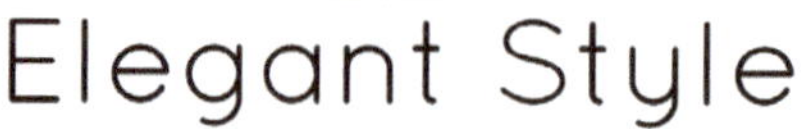

Elegant Style

Elegant style always like to look neat, distinguished, and refined. They show authority and an elevated position in society. Their messages are of success and perfection, besides that they are always well dressed according to the occasion. The risk is to seem conceited or arrogant.

Just as the natural style prefers comfort, the elegant prefers quality. For this reason they are saving people, because they know that investing in the quality of their clothes is something important. This style is the most difficult to achieve, because all the time they must be attentive to the details.

The designs that they prefer are formal, with straight lines, and that fit the body perfectly. Hardly any prints are used, unless they're very small, almost imperceptible. The colors used are: black, white, grey. They also used solid and sober colors that combine with each other.

Haircut is controlled, from medium to short and timeless. Makeup is always present in women, and must be perfectly done, without any mistake. Accessories are neither very large, nor very small, but suitable for the complexion of the person.

I recommend you keep it up, you are on the right track. The only thing I would say is that you have more fun with the combination of garments, of course without losing your essence.

Celebrities with elegant style: Tom Ford and Kate Middleton

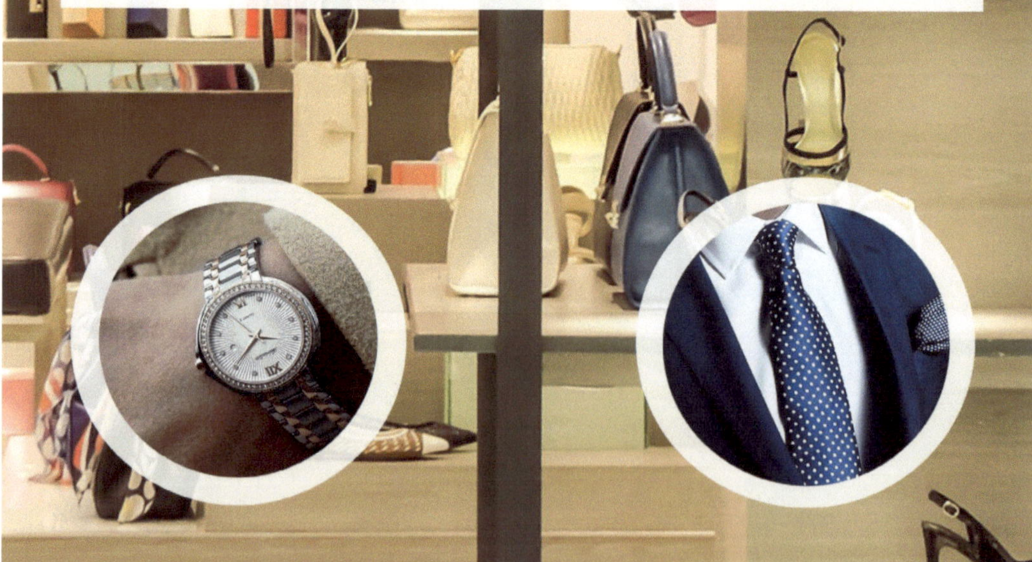

Romantic Style

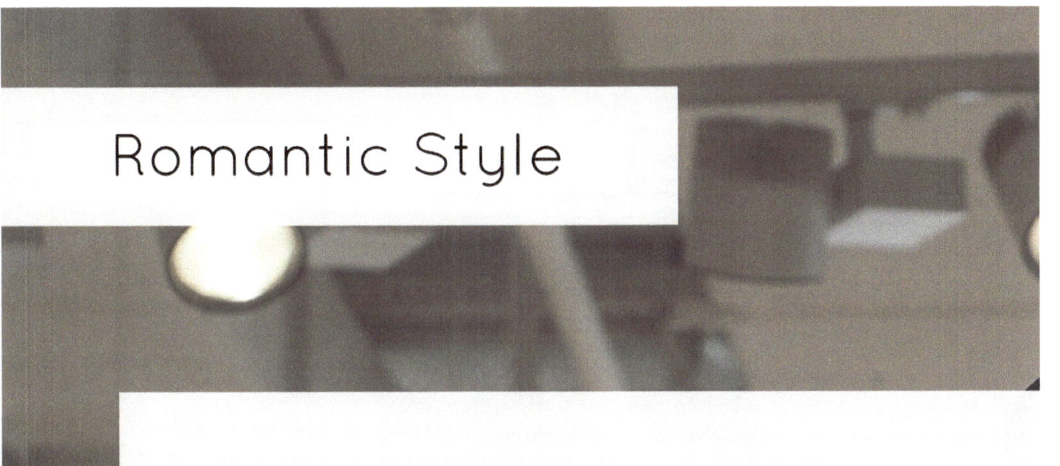

People with romantic style often have many friends, because they inspire confidence and cordiality. They show kindness, empathy, peace, etc. What more can they ask for? Maybe you are relating this style to something very sweet or cheesy, but it is not. Although the risk is to look cheesy, or naïve, it has many more features.

They tend to be gentle, tender, and charming people. Just as the elegant style prefers quality, the romantic style prefers kindness. In the case of women, they always want to look more feminine. The colors they love the most are pastels, nothing too strong or flashy.

Women prefer dresses with free fall, lace, and classics. Men prefer relaxed lines and less structure. Both like light textures, such as rayon, velvet, and silk.

Haircut goes from medium to long, with waves, and hair highlights. Makeup carries pastel tones, is very sweet, and with emphasize eyelashes. Accessories are sets that combine with each other, very feminine, simple, and with figurative touches.

My recommendation is that you keep producing your style as you do, because you will project confidence and cordiality. Just do not abuse the cheesy, so you don't fall for the risk.

Celebrities with romantic style: Ryan Gosling and Taylor Swift

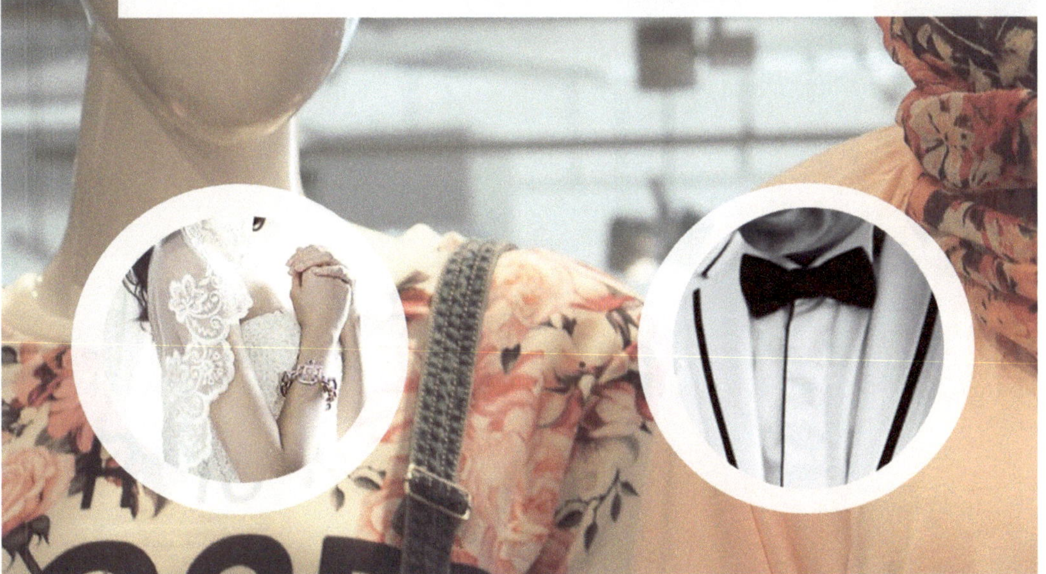

Seductive Style

Surely many people tell you that you are sexy, you are very attractive to others. They prefer good fit, rather than comfort. Just be careful because you may look a little indecent.

You like outfits that highlight your body, as well as risky and intense designs with contrasting combinations. Hairstyle can be wavy or straight, from medium to long, and with lots of volume. Makeup is sensual and it is made with precision, lips stand out.

In men, facial hair is present, very well groomed and defined. Accessories are striking and large. Some people who have seductive style like tattoos.

My recommendation is to leave space for moderation inside your closet, that way you would not fall into the risk of looking indecent. Beware of maxi necklines or mini skirts, remember that less is more in terms of elegance. Try to make your outfits look more discreet and elegant, of course without losing your essence.

Celebrities with seductive style: David Beckham and Megan Fox

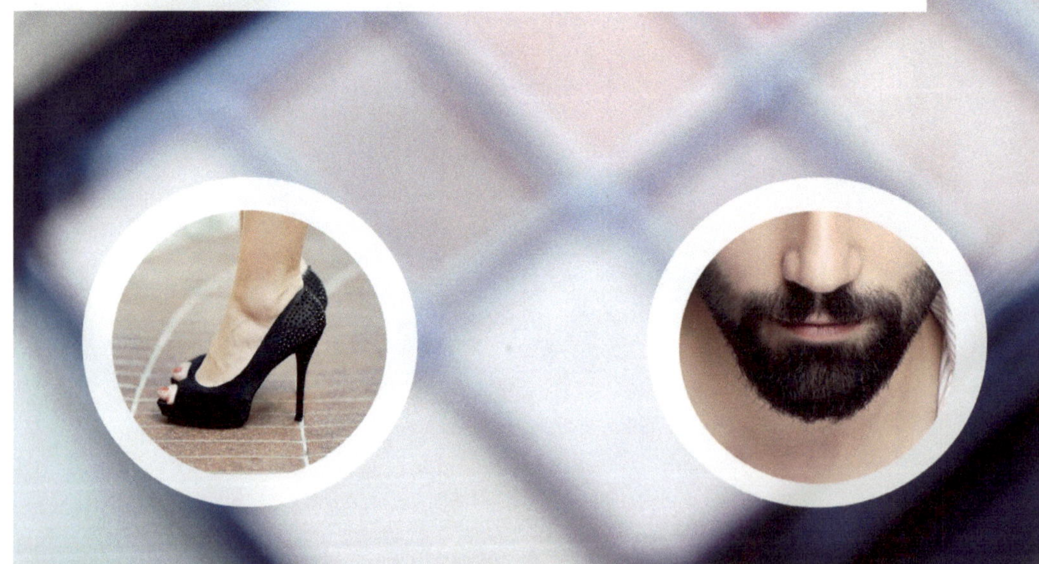

Creative Style

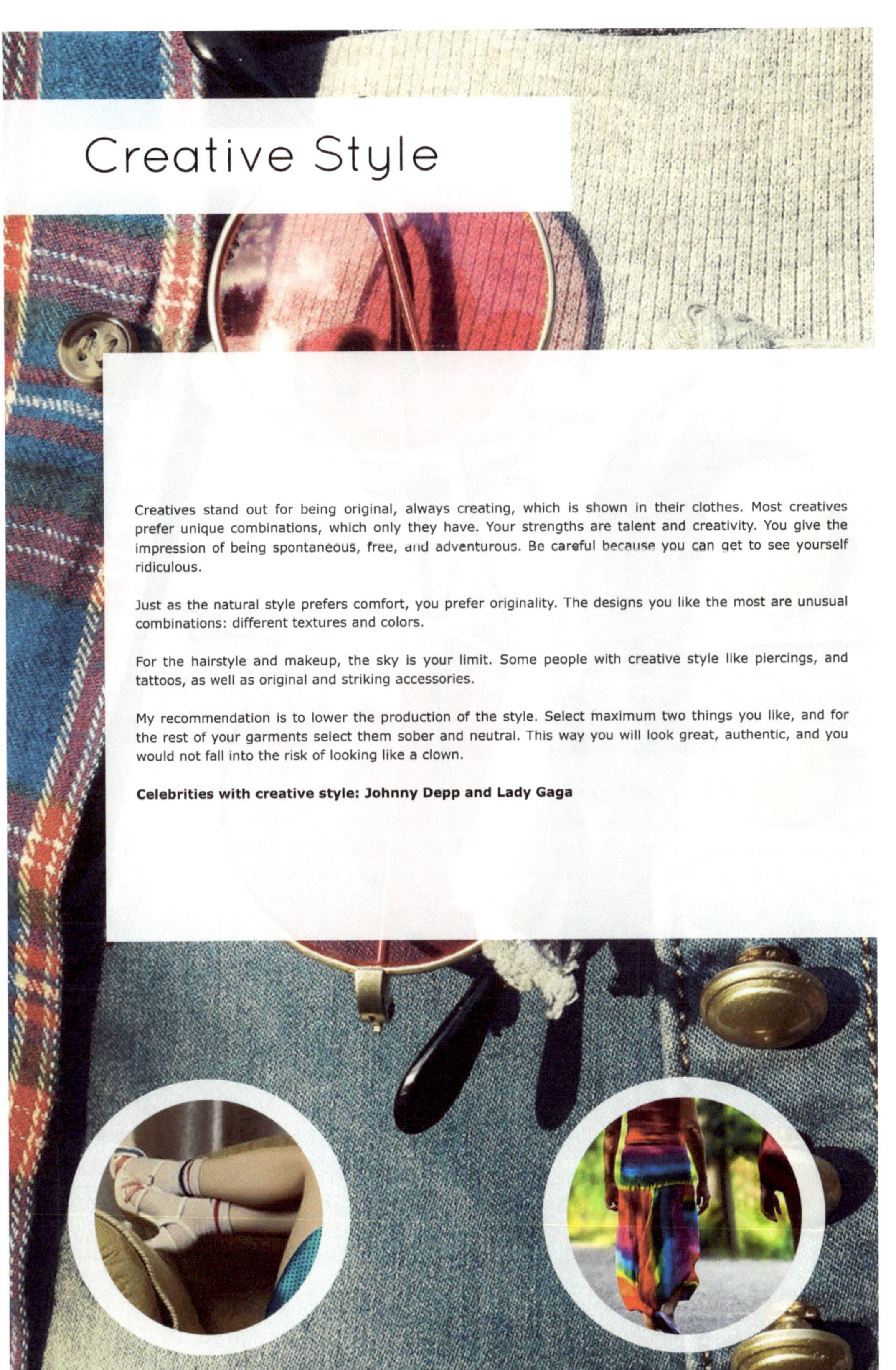

Creatives stand out for being original, always creating, which is shown in their clothes. Most creatives prefer unique combinations, which only they have. Your strengths are talent and creativity. You give the impression of being spontaneous, free, and adventurous. Be careful because you can get to see yourself ridiculous.

Just as the natural style prefers comfort, you prefer originality. The designs you like the most are unusual combinations: different textures and colors.

For the hairstyle and makeup, the sky is your limit. Some people with creative style like piercings, and tattoos, as well as original and striking accessories.

My recommendation is to lower the production of the style. Select maximum two things you like, and for the rest of your garments select them sober and neutral. This way you will look great, authentic, and you would not fall into the risk of looking like a clown.

Celebrities with creative style: Johnny Depp and Lady Gaga

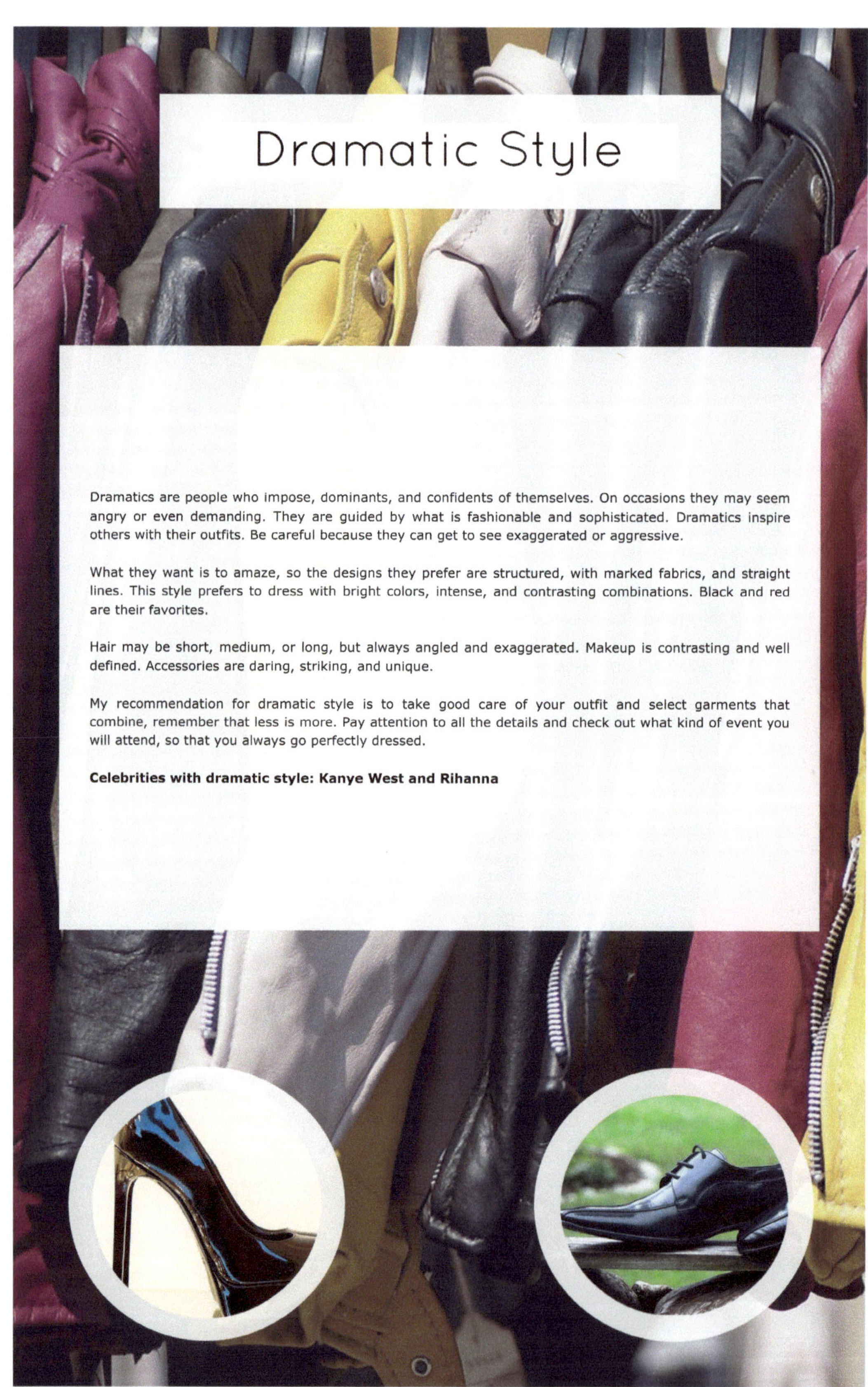

Dramatic Style

Dramatics are people who impose, dominants, and confidents of themselves. On occasions they may seem angry or even demanding. They are guided by what is fashionable and sophisticated. Dramatics inspire others with their outfits. Be careful because they can get to see exaggerated or aggressive.

What they want is to amaze, so the designs they prefer are structured, with marked fabrics, and straight lines. This style prefers to dress with bright colors, intense, and contrasting combinations. Black and red are their favorites.

Hair may be short, medium, or long, but always angled and exaggerated. Makeup is contrasting and well defined. Accessories are daring, striking, and unique.

My recommendation for dramatic style is to take good care of your outfit and select garments that combine, remember that less is more. Pay attention to all the details and check out what kind of event you will attend, so that you always go perfectly dressed.

Celebrities with dramatic style: Kanye West and Rihanna

I am sure you identify yourself with the phrase "I have nothing to wear." I bet your closet is full, and it does not fit a single item anymore. What happens is that you do not feel comfortable with your clothes, maybe they are very old fabrics or your body has changed. Maybe those colors do not highlight your beauty, or maybe, or maybe, or maybe.

That is why this profession is so quoted nowadays, people want to feel good and look radiant. And they want the whole process to be fast, cheap, and with good results.

I have great news, a basic and versatile wardrobe, requires only 20 garments. That is where my work comes in, because you have to strategically select the clothes so that they all combine and always look spectacular.

One of my strategies is to have neutral clothes, but also your favorites, some that make you stand out. The favorites will call the attention, and the neutral ones you can use them again and again, without looking like a photograph.

I invite you to buy your favorite garments, those that make you feel unique. Combine them and highlight your style to the fullest!

Now that I will tell you all the clothes you need for your wardrobe, you will probably wonder how to combine them. So here I leave you some ideas. I assure you this is the more creative part and your imagination is the limit.

Let's have some fun!

Make the most of your garments

- 1 jacket or coat in dark colors.
- 1 dark-colored sweater with buttons.
- 2 white shirts.
- 1 solid-colored shirt.
- 3 solid and neutral colored T-shirts.
- 2 suits, one dark blue, and another dark grey.
- 3 formal trousers: black, solid-colored and dark grey.
- 1 black belt on one side, and coffee or blue on the other side.
- 2 ties.
- 1 pair of jeans, without washes or holes, neutral, and smooth.
- 1 pair of black and formal shoes.
- 1 pair of suede brown shoes.
- 1 casual white tennis.

Some ideas to combine your wardrobe (men):

- To go to the movies with your friends, combine your jeans with a colored shirt and white tennis.

- Wear jeans with a colored shirt and brown shoes, for a Friday at the office.

- For a brunch with your family, combine the jeans with a white shirt and the dark sweater. Brown shoes will look great.

- Khakis with white shirt, reversible coffee belt, a raincoat, and brown shoes will look great for a day of meetings in the Office.

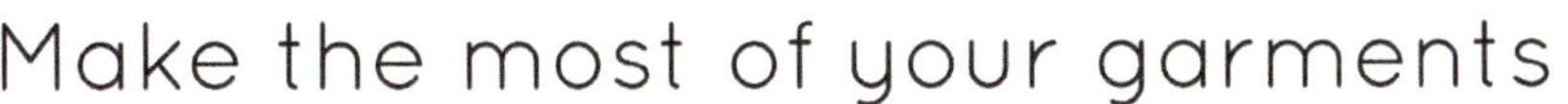

Make the most of your garments

- 1 jacket or coat in dark colors.
- 1 dark-colored sweater with buttons.
- 2 white shirts.
- 1 solid-colored shirt.
- 4 solid and neutral colored blouses.
- 3 formal trousers, one black, one clear, and one dark grey.
- 1 black belt on one side, and coffee or blue on the other.
- 2 skirts at knee height.
- 1 black dress at knee height.
- 1 pair of jeans, without washes or holes, neutral, and smooth.
- 1 pair of closed-toe shoes, black, and others in brown color.
- 1 pair of open-heeled shoes, black, and others in brown color.
- 1 pair of black boots and one of low shoes "flats".

Some ideas to combine your wardrobe (women):

- For work or a formal event, white shirts look good with black pants and black shoes.

- For family meals choose jeans, white shirt, and open-toed shoes.

- For an event with your friends, wear your favorite skirt with a white shirt, and combine it with the brown open shoes.

- When having a brunch with your friends, combine the pair of jeans with your favorite blouse, and the brown closed heels.

- For a lazy day, combine your jeans and low shoes with the black sweater, along with your favorite blouse.

- For a Friday at the office, combine your jeans with the white shirt, black heels, and a color bag.

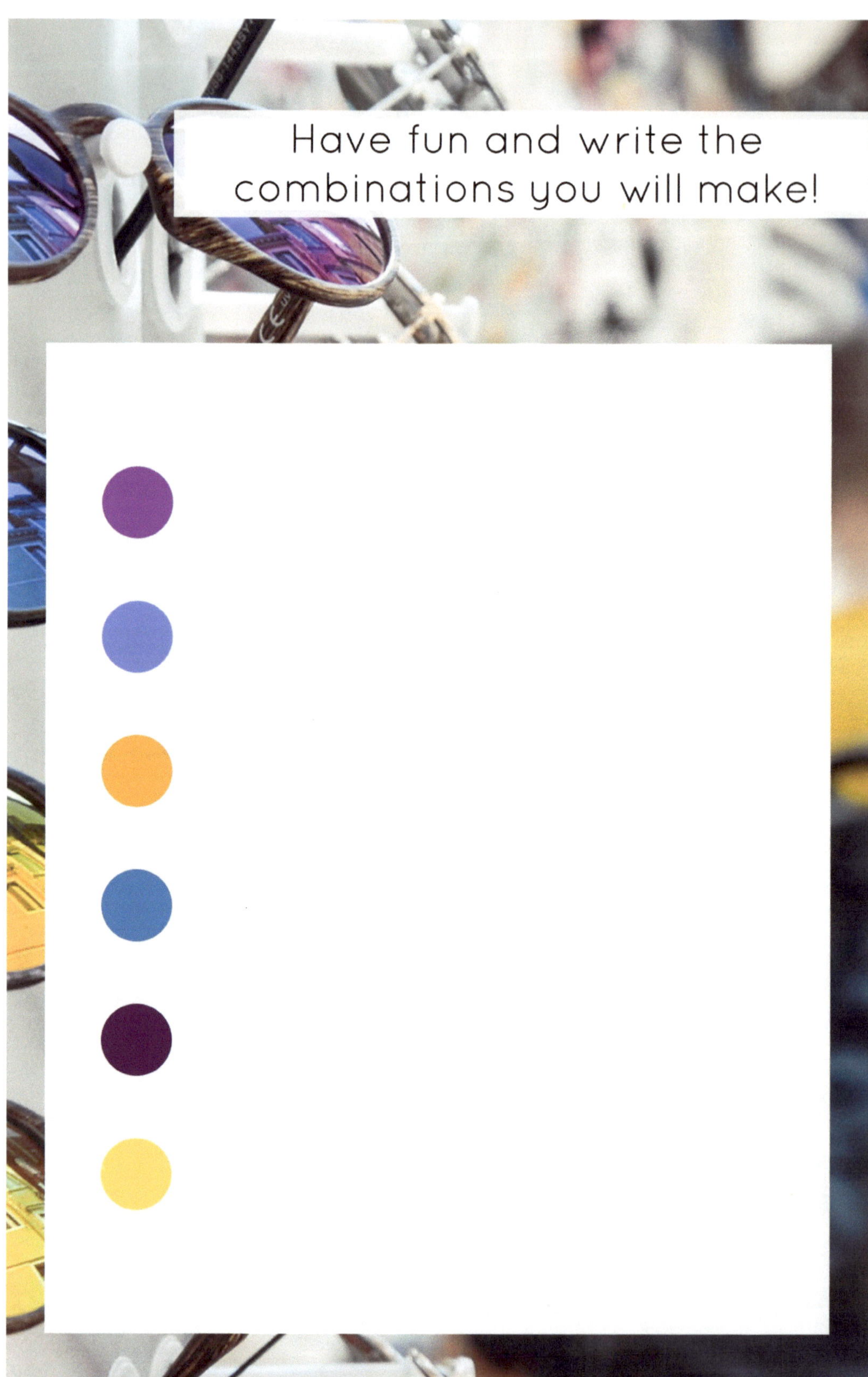

Have fun and write the
combinations you will make!

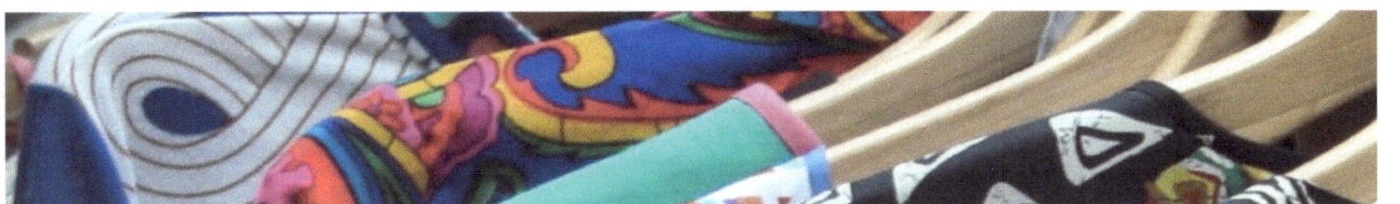

Neither fruits, nor geometric figures

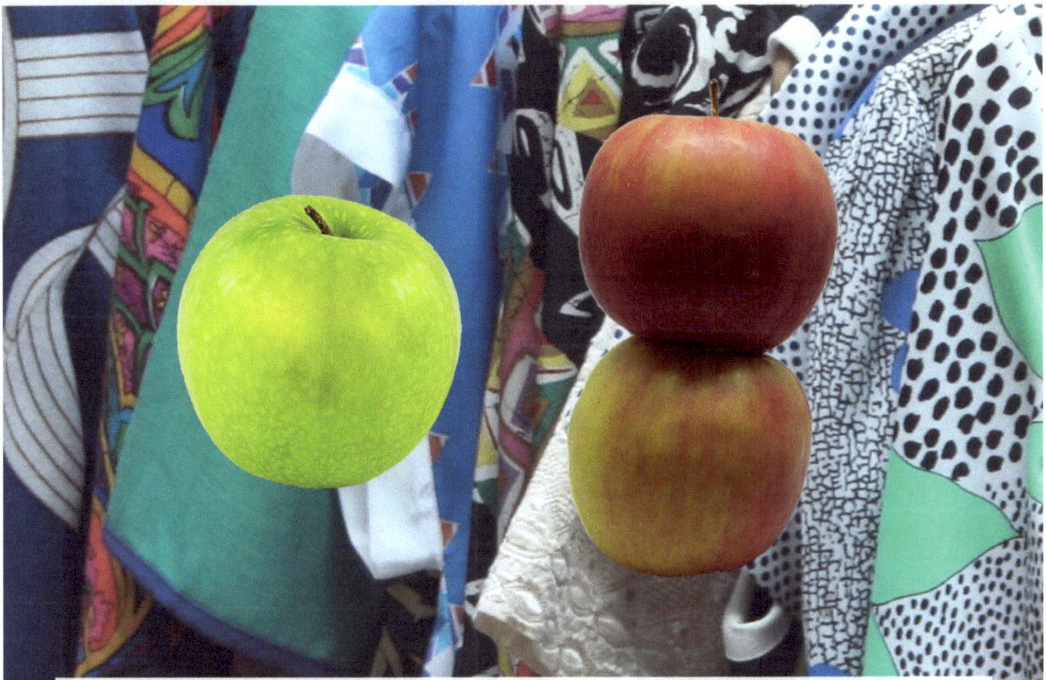

There is a conflict within me to name this topic. Many colleagues call the body shapes with fruit names. For example: apple or pear. Others, classify them with cutlery names, such as: knife or spoon. And many others prefer to refer to geometric shapes, such as: circle or triangle.

But for me a body goes far beyond that, because we are all completely and absolutely different. These parameters serve to pigeonhole body types and provide general recommendations. Some may work, but what actually works is when the image consultant analyzes every measurement of your body in detail. That is how she or he can determine the recommendations that are just for you.

In order for you to have these services, you will need to go with an image consultant. Only she or he can give you personalized recommendations. I am sure you will love the results.

This is a very personal science, no generalizations.

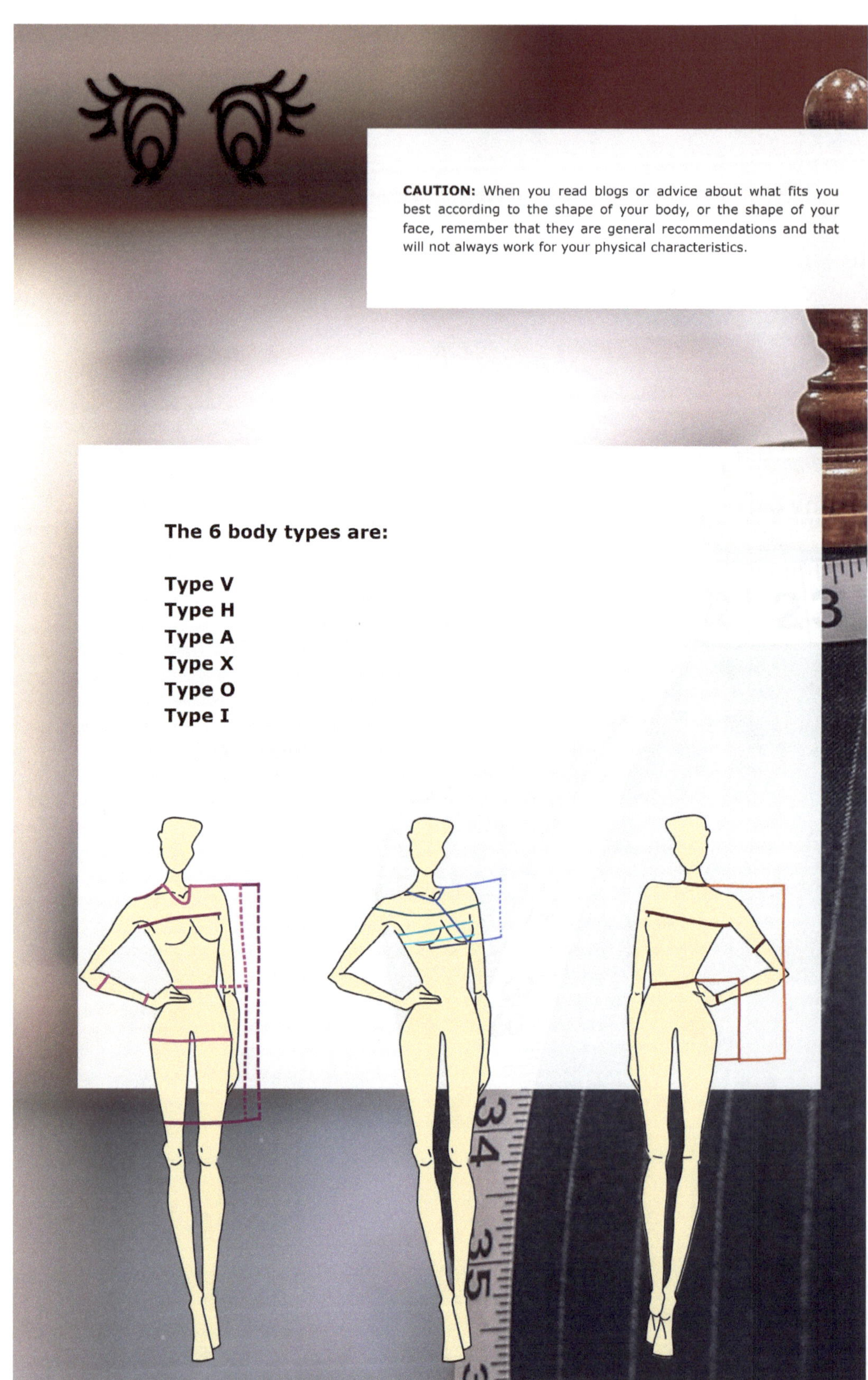

CAUTION: When you read blogs or advice about what fits you best according to the shape of your body, or the shape of your face, remember that they are general recommendations and that will not always work for your physical characteristics.

The 6 body types are:

Type V
Type H
Type A
Type X
Type O
Type I

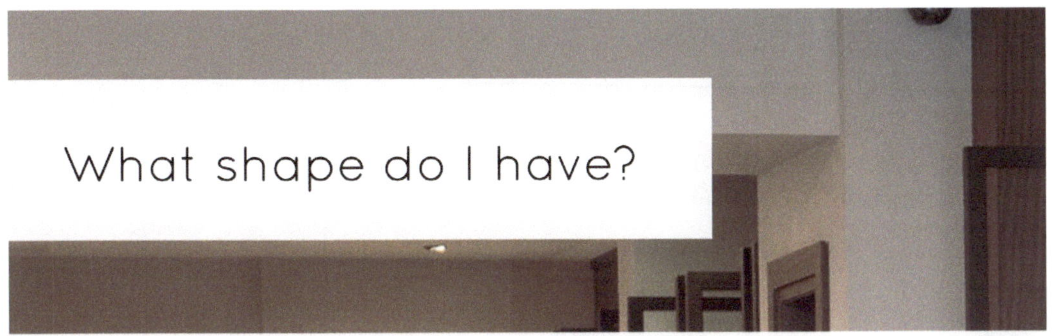

What shape do I have?

For you to know what body shape you have, I recommend you to take a picture of your whole body with tight clothes, then print it. Then, analyze what letter looks more like your body. When you are done reading all the explanations of the body types, decide what type of body is yours. Finally, draw the letter on the picture, above your body.

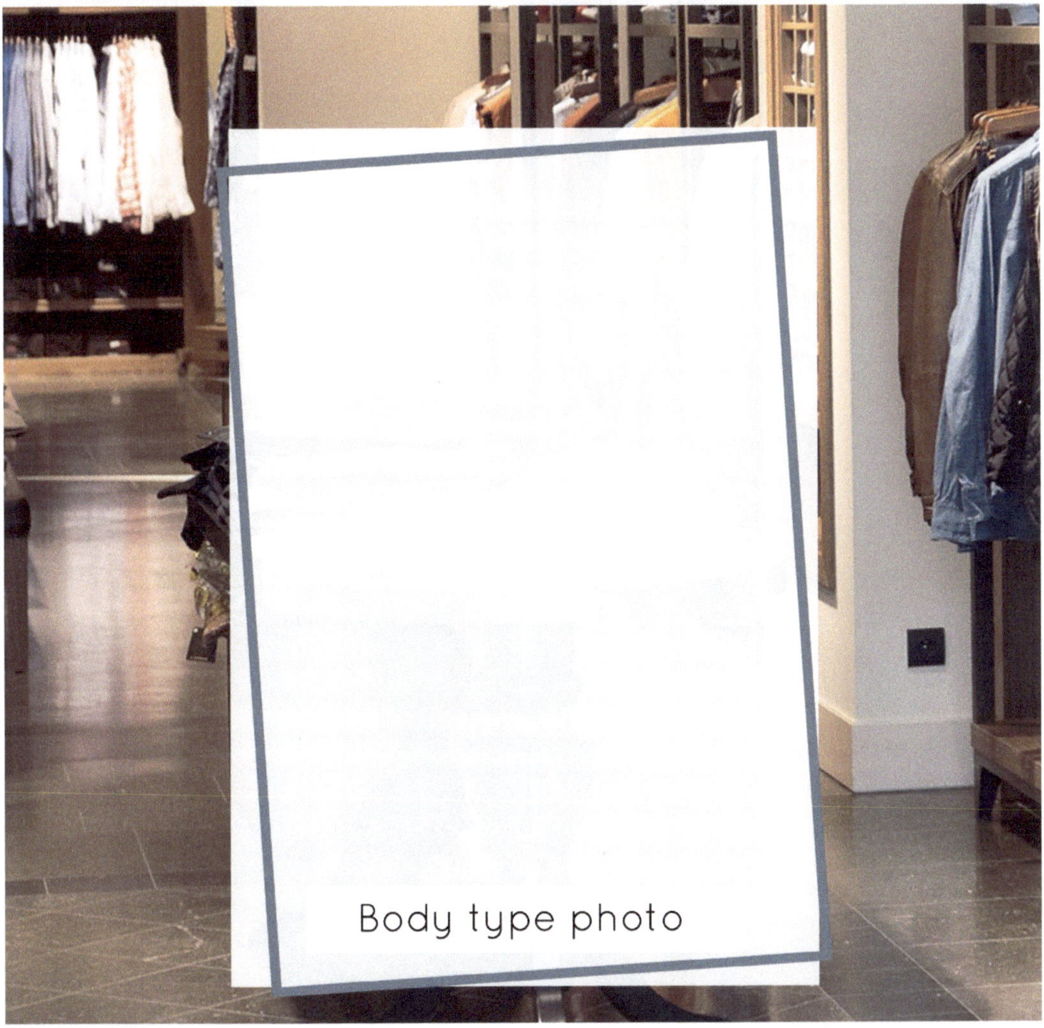

Body type photo

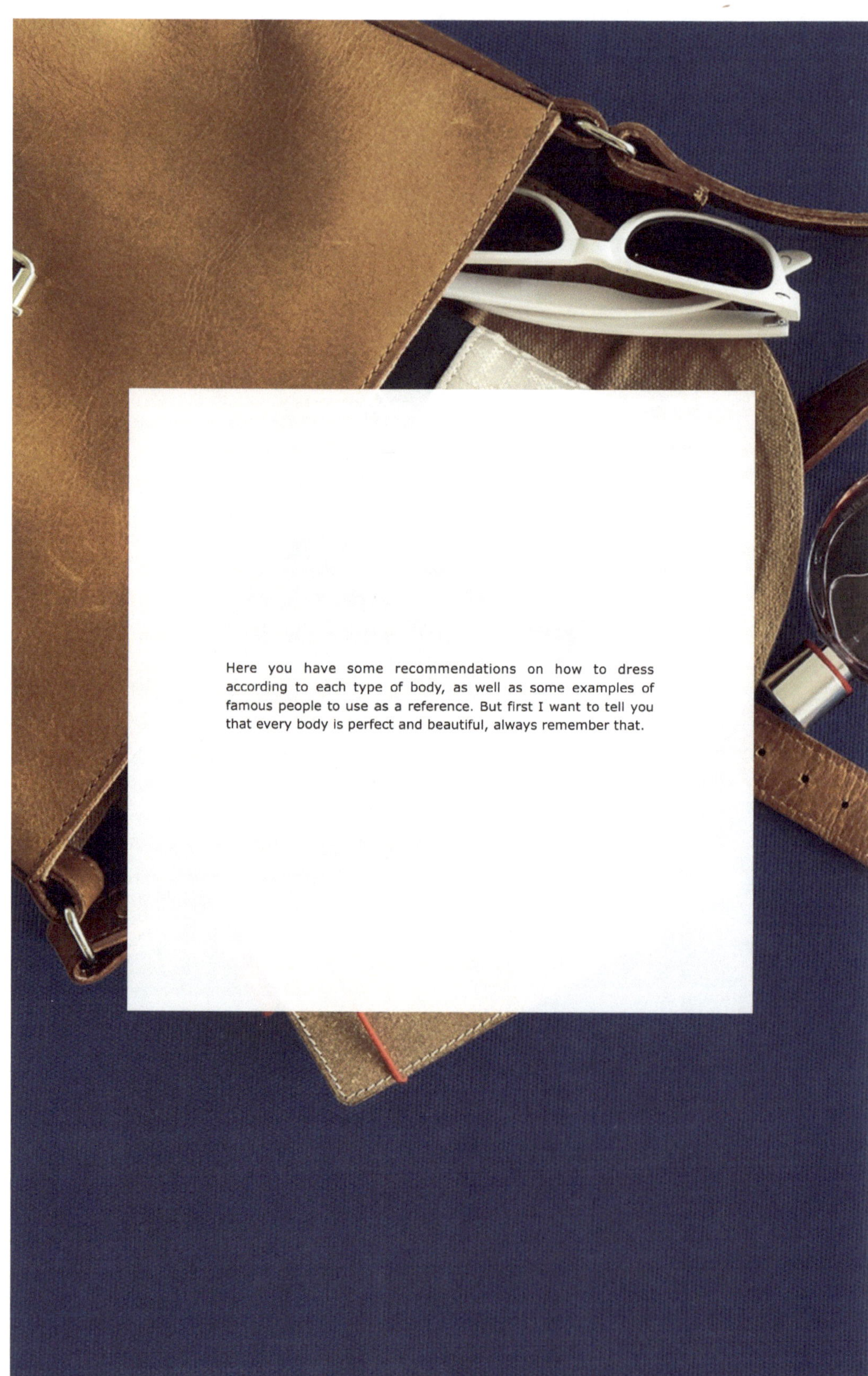

Here you have some recommendations on how to dress according to each type of body, as well as some examples of famous people to use as a reference. But first I want to tell you that every body is perfect and beautiful, always remember that.

Body shape type V

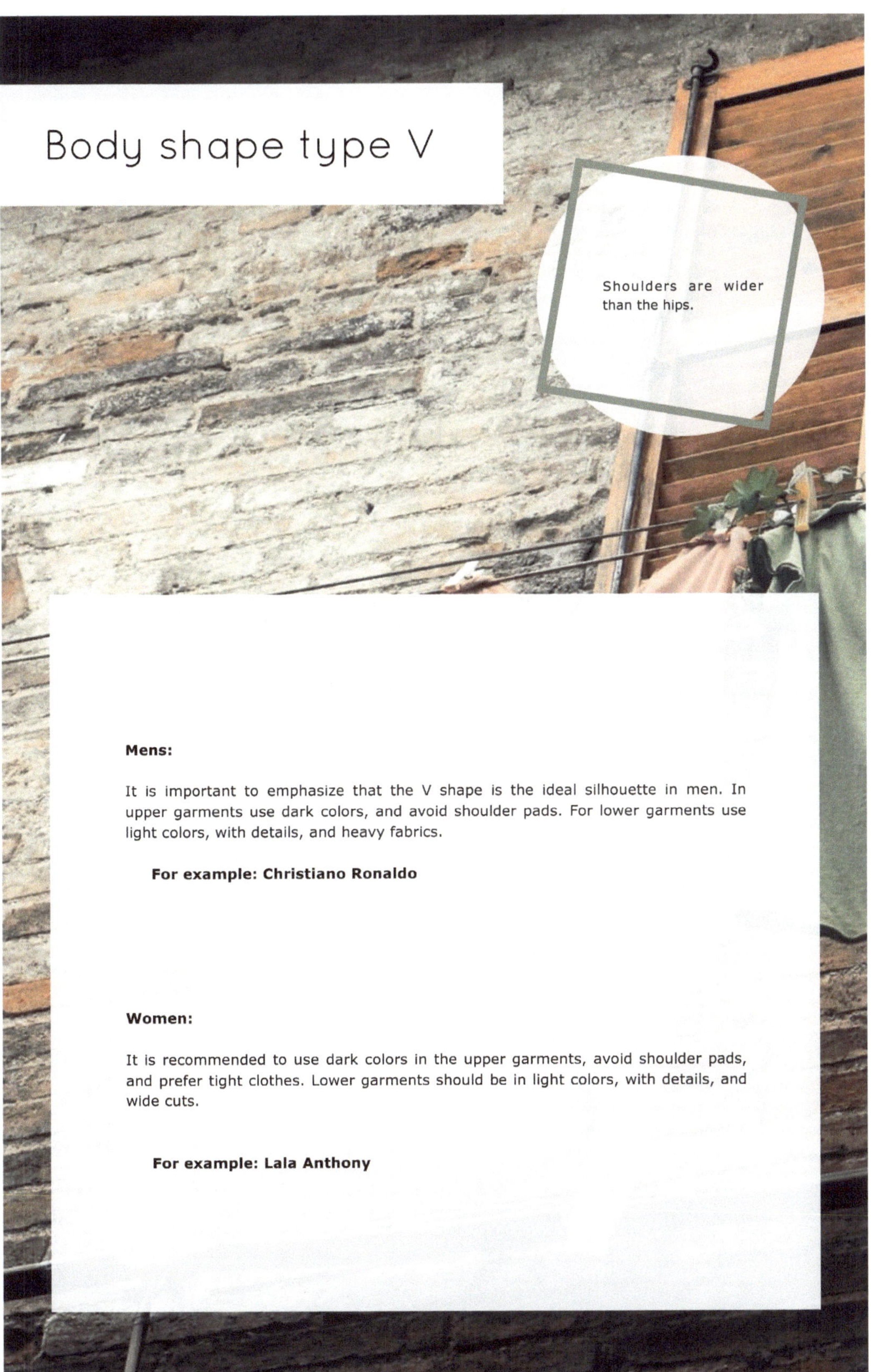

Mens:

It is important to emphasize that the V shape is the ideal silhouette in men. In upper garments use dark colors, and avoid shoulder pads. For lower garments use light colors, with details, and heavy fabrics.

For example: Christiano Ronaldo

Women:

It is recommended to use dark colors in the upper garments, avoid shoulder pads, and prefer tight clothes. Lower garments should be in light colors, with details, and wide cuts.

For example: Lala Anthony

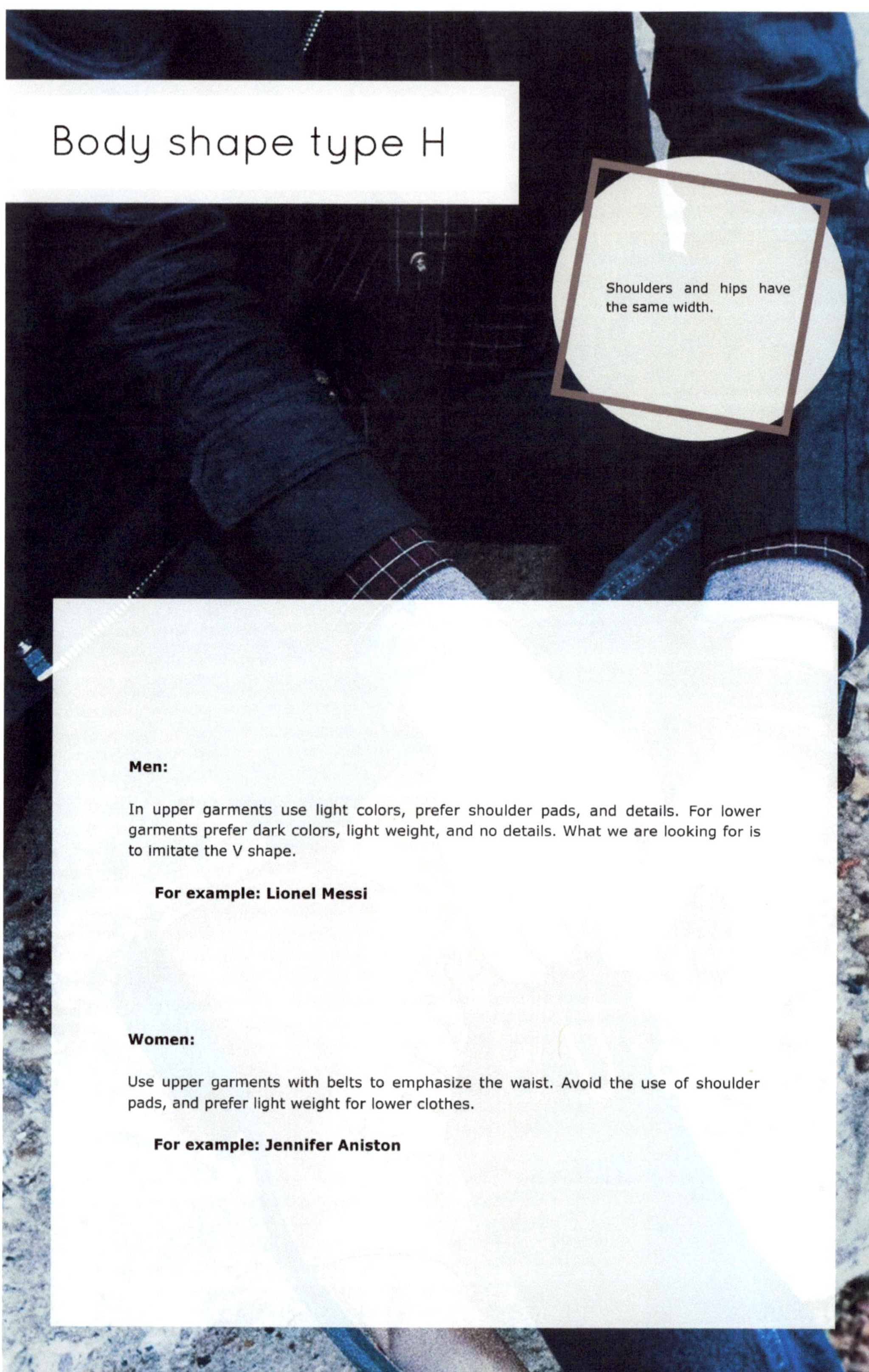

Body shape type H

Shoulders and hips have the same width.

Men:

In upper garments use light colors, prefer shoulder pads, and details. For lower garments prefer dark colors, light weight, and no details. What we are looking for is to imitate the V shape.

For example: Lionel Messi

Women:

Use upper garments with belts to emphasize the waist. Avoid the use of shoulder pads, and prefer light weight for lower clothes.

For example: Jennifer Aniston

Body shape type A

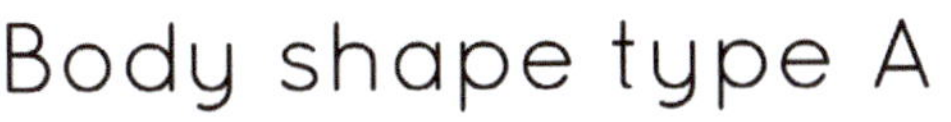

Hips are wider than the shoulders.

Men:

The upper garments must be light-colored, with details, and horizontal designs. For the lower clothes, the colors will be dark, and without details.

For example: Adam Sandler

Women:

Wear top garments in light colors, with details, and heavy fabrics. For the lower garments choose dark colors, and light fabrics. Lower clothes should be adjusted.

For example: Alicia Keys

Body shape type X

Men:

There is no such body type in men.

Women:

It is the ideal body for women, so they can dress as they want to. It is recommended to emphasize the waist in order to maintain a harmonious and balanced body. When there are curves in the body, the body type is called 8 instead of X. Both have the same characteristics, only that 8 is more rounded.

For example: Heidi Klum or Beyoncé

Body shape type O

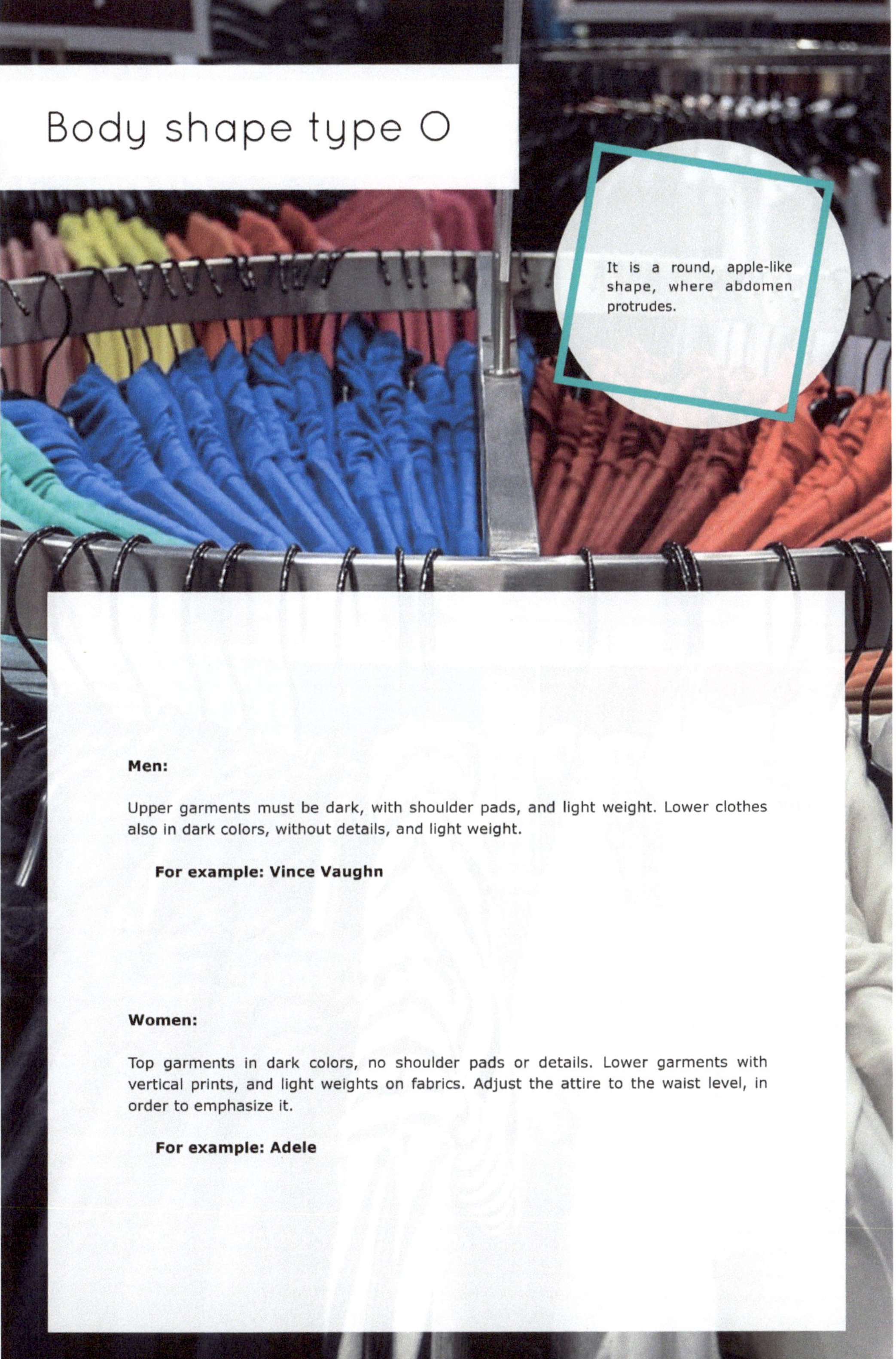

It is a round, apple-like shape, where abdomen protrudes.

Men:

Upper garments must be dark, with shoulder pads, and light weight. Lower clothes also in dark colors, without details, and light weight.

For example: Vince Vaughn

Women:

Top garments in dark colors, no shoulder pads or details. Lower garments with vertical prints, and light weights on fabrics. Adjust the attire to the waist level, in order to emphasize it.

For example: Adele

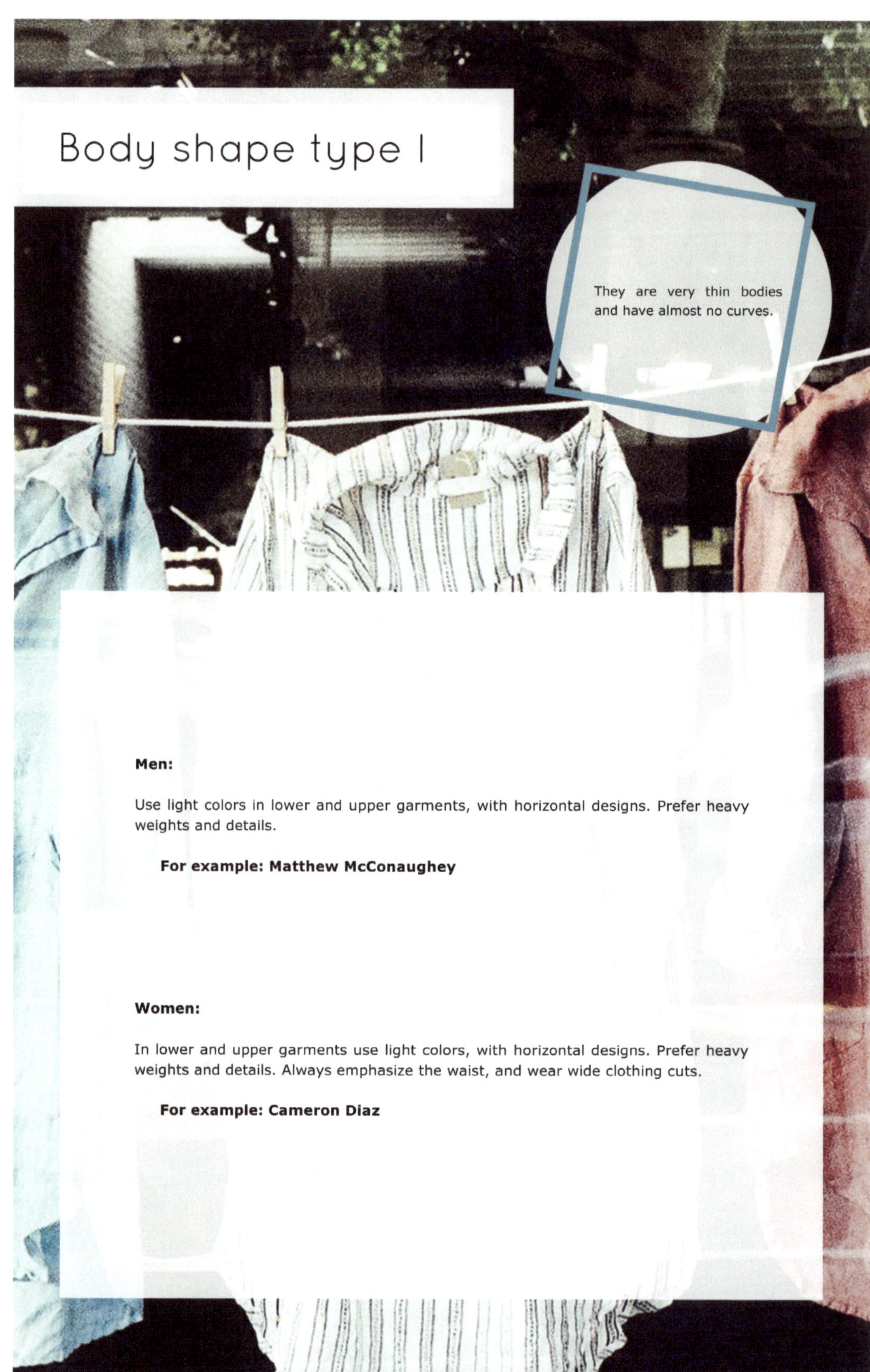

Body shape type I

Men:

Use light colors in lower and upper garments, with horizontal designs. Prefer heavy weights and details.

For example: Matthew McConaughey

Women:

In lower and upper garments use light colors, with horizontal designs. Prefer heavy weights and details. Always emphasize the waist, and wear wide clothing cuts.

For example: Cameron Diaz

To the party or to the office?

You wake up at 7 in the morning, then you prepare your breakfast, then you take a shower, finally you dress up and go out to conquer the day.

The morning is sunny and warm, everything goes great with your outfit, because you wear shorts and a short-sleeved shirt. But in the afternoon the weather changes dramatically and it starts to rain. Your outfit is not longer the best, now you are cold and the rain soaks you. Your outfit is no good anymore.

Have you heard this story?

Or maybe you identify more with the next scenario.

You dressed up perfectly well for your cousin's baptism, because you think it will be in a very elegant and closed room. So you decided to wear a dress with stilettos, because you will look very elegant and according to the occasion. But when you arrive to the event you realize that the location is the opposite of what you thought, it is in an outdoor garden.

Your perfect outfit just failed. The heels are buried in the grass, you are already sweating. And as if that were not enough, you already have a red face because of the sun.

Has this happened to you, or do you know someone who has gone through this?

Surely these scenarios sound familiar, as people are not used to check important details to always be well dressed at events. But do not worry, now we will see what you should do before attending an event, so that you always look great.

Rules before
leaving your house

1

Check the weather. Make sure you know if it will be cold, hot, rainy, etc.

2

Confirm the time of the event. It is very different to dress up for an event that will be during the day, than for one that will be at night.

3

Check the location of the event. If it will be in a garden, in a lounge, in a church, on the beach, etc. It is not the same to dress up for going to the church, than for going to the beach.

To always look good and consistent, you must follow the three rules that we just mentioned.

Now, I am going to give you some examples of dress codes, so you know how you should be dressed at different events.

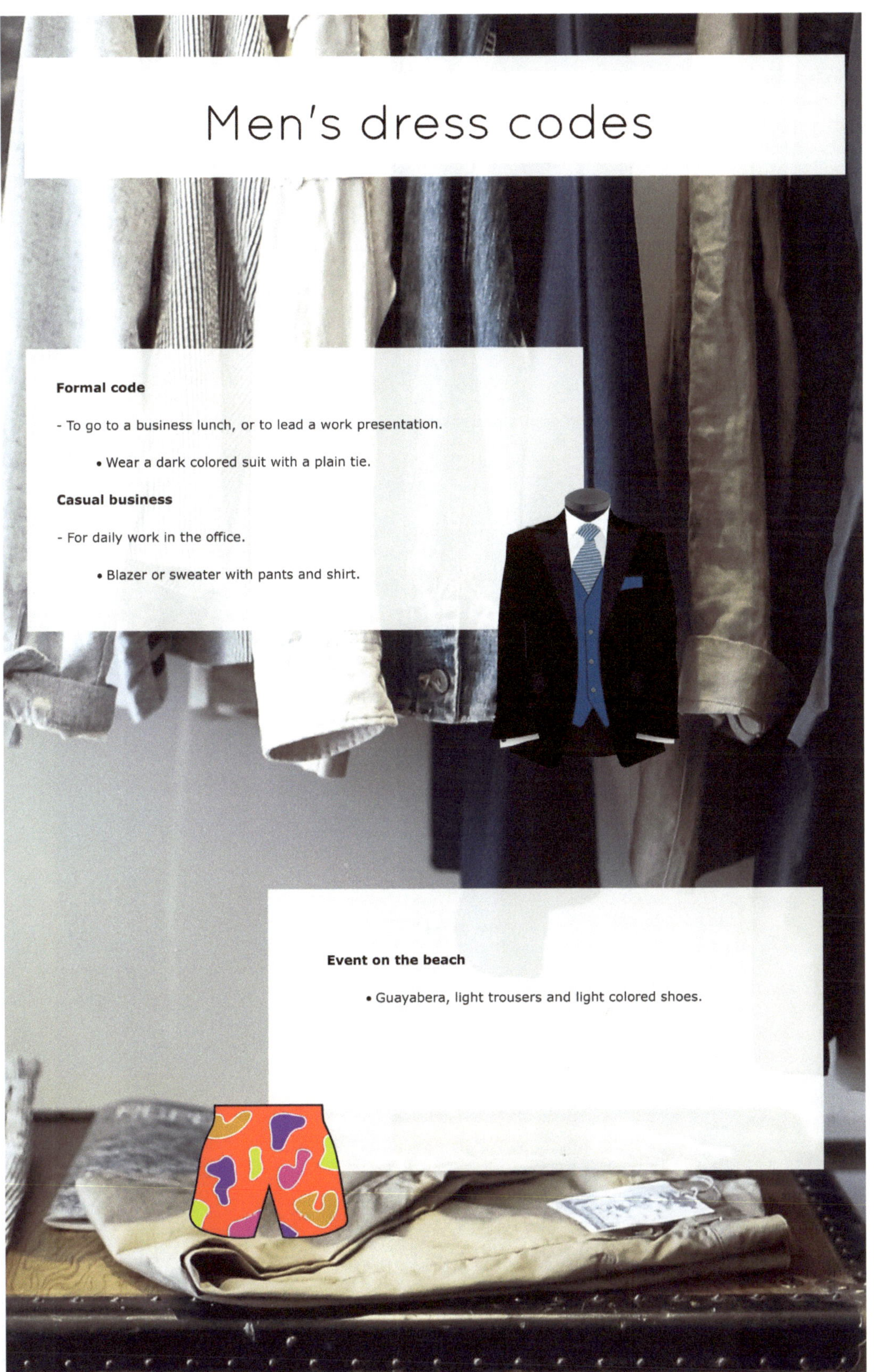

Men's dress codes

Formal code

- To go to a business lunch, or to lead a work presentation.

  • Wear a dark colored suit with a plain tie.

Casual business

- For daily work in the office.

  • Blazer or sweater with pants and shirt.

Event on the beach

  • Guayabera, light trousers and light colored shoes.

Women's dress codes

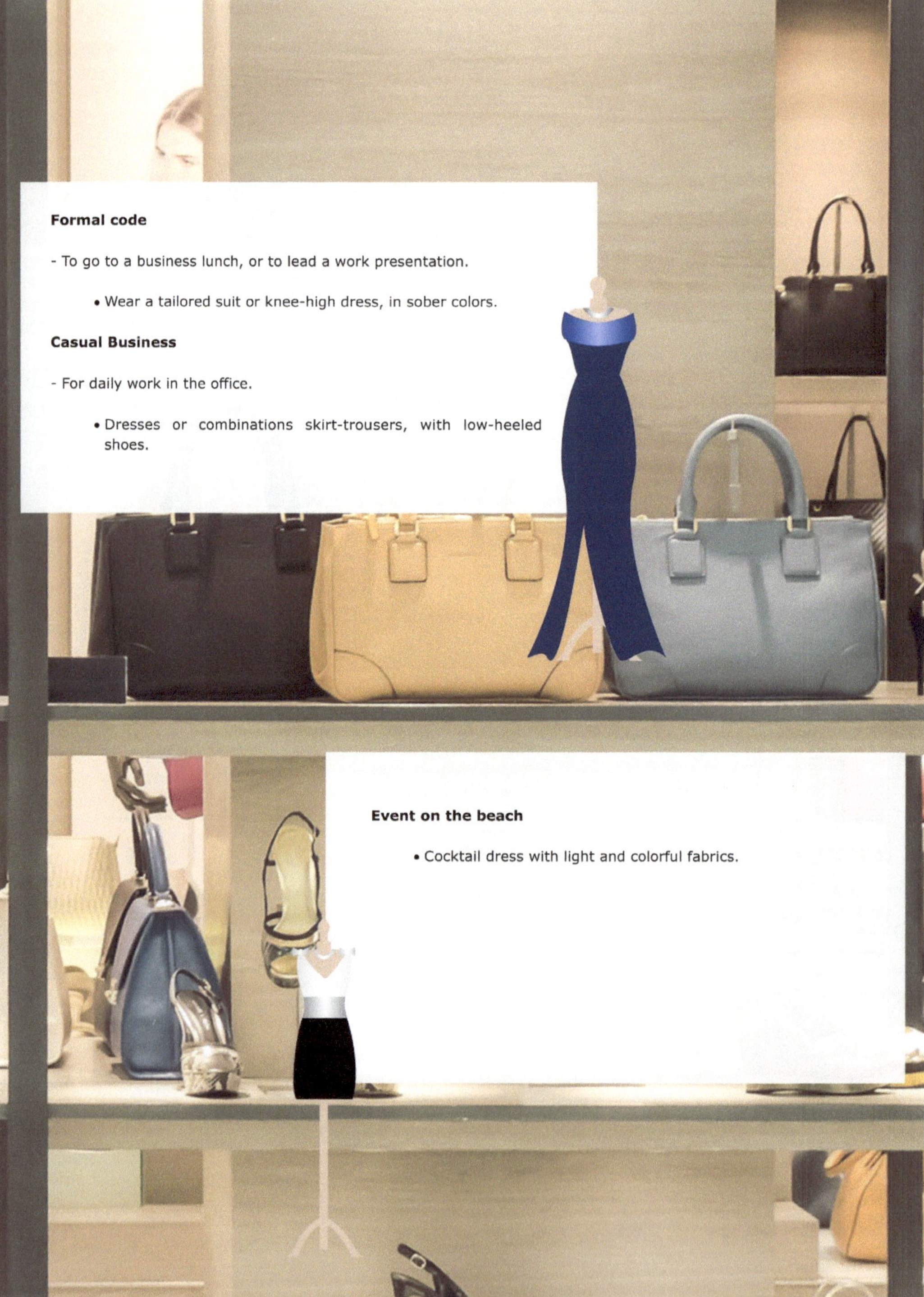

Grandma's Advice

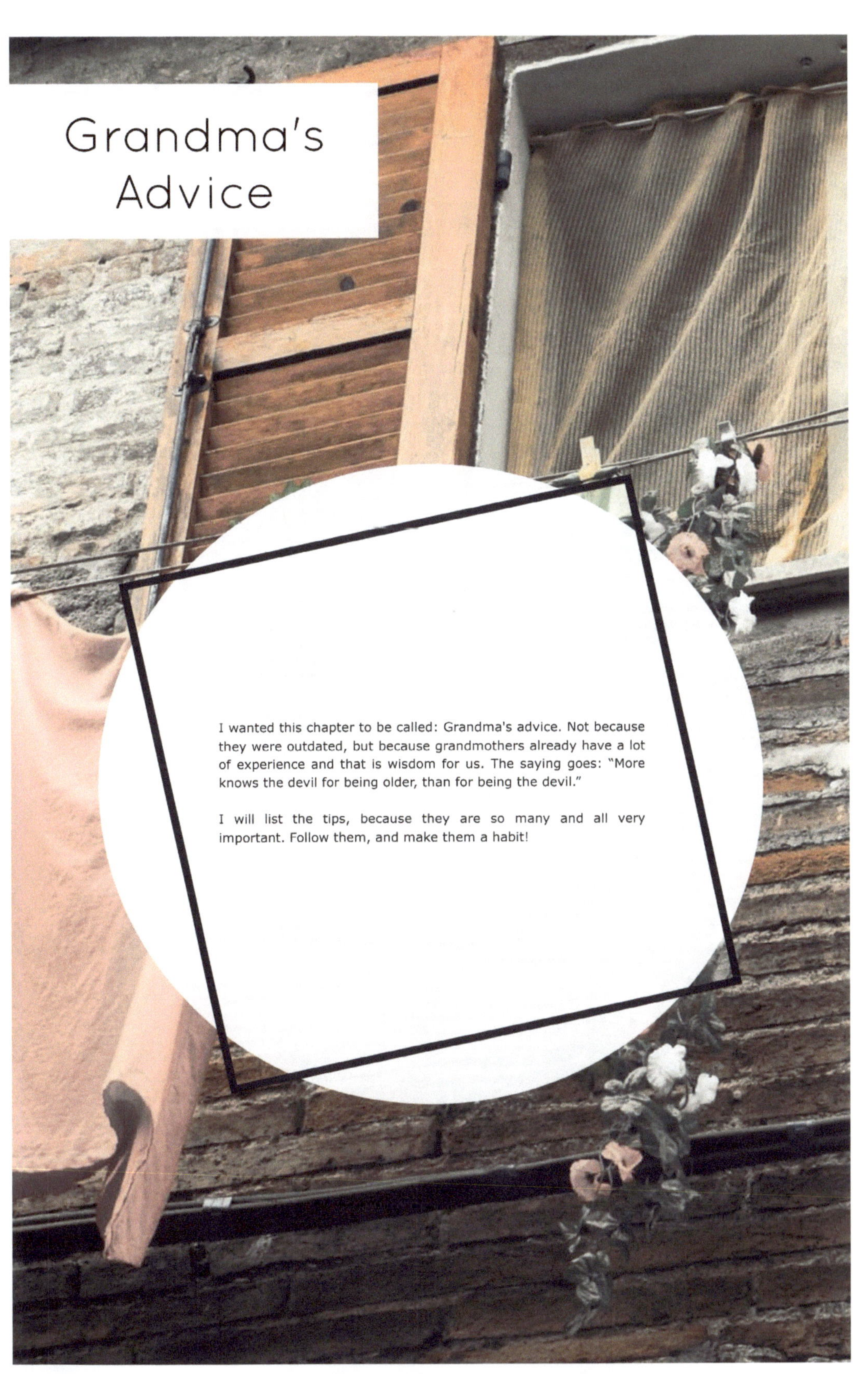

I wanted this chapter to be called: Grandma's advice. Not because they were outdated, but because grandmothers already have a lot of experience and that is wisdom for us. The saying goes: "More knows the devil for being older, than for being the devil."

I will list the tips, because they are so many and all very important. Follow them, and make them a habit!

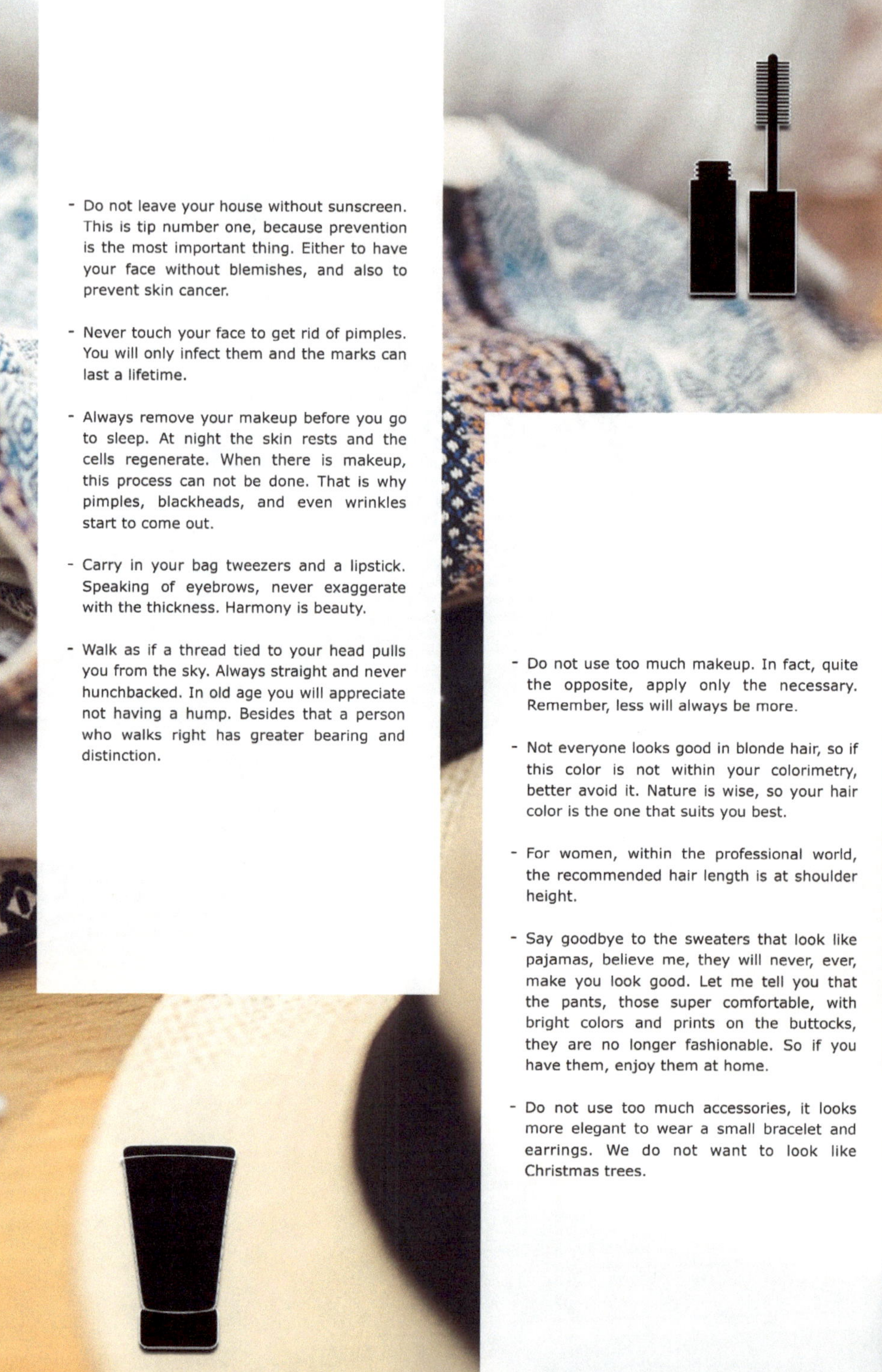

- Do not leave your house without sunscreen. This is tip number one, because prevention is the most important thing. Either to have your face without blemishes, and also to prevent skin cancer.

- Never touch your face to get rid of pimples. You will only infect them and the marks can last a lifetime.

- Always remove your makeup before you go to sleep. At night the skin rests and the cells regenerate. When there is makeup, this process can not be done. That is why pimples, blackheads, and even wrinkles start to come out.

- Carry in your bag tweezers and a lipstick. Speaking of eyebrows, never exaggerate with the thickness. Harmony is beauty.

- Walk as if a thread tied to your head pulls you from the sky. Always straight and never hunchbacked. In old age you will appreciate not having a hump. Besides that a person who walks right has greater bearing and distinction.

- Do not use too much makeup. In fact, quite the opposite, apply only the necessary. Remember, less will always be more.

- Not everyone looks good in blonde hair, so if this color is not within your colorimetry, better avoid it. Nature is wise, so your hair color is the one that suits you best.

- For women, within the professional world, the recommended hair length is at shoulder height.

- Say goodbye to the sweaters that look like pajamas, believe me, they will never, ever, make you look good. Let me tell you that the pants, those super comfortable, with bright colors and prints on the buttocks, they are no longer fashionable. So if you have them, enjoy them at home.

- Do not use too much accessories, it looks more elegant to wear a small bracelet and earrings. We do not want to look like Christmas trees.

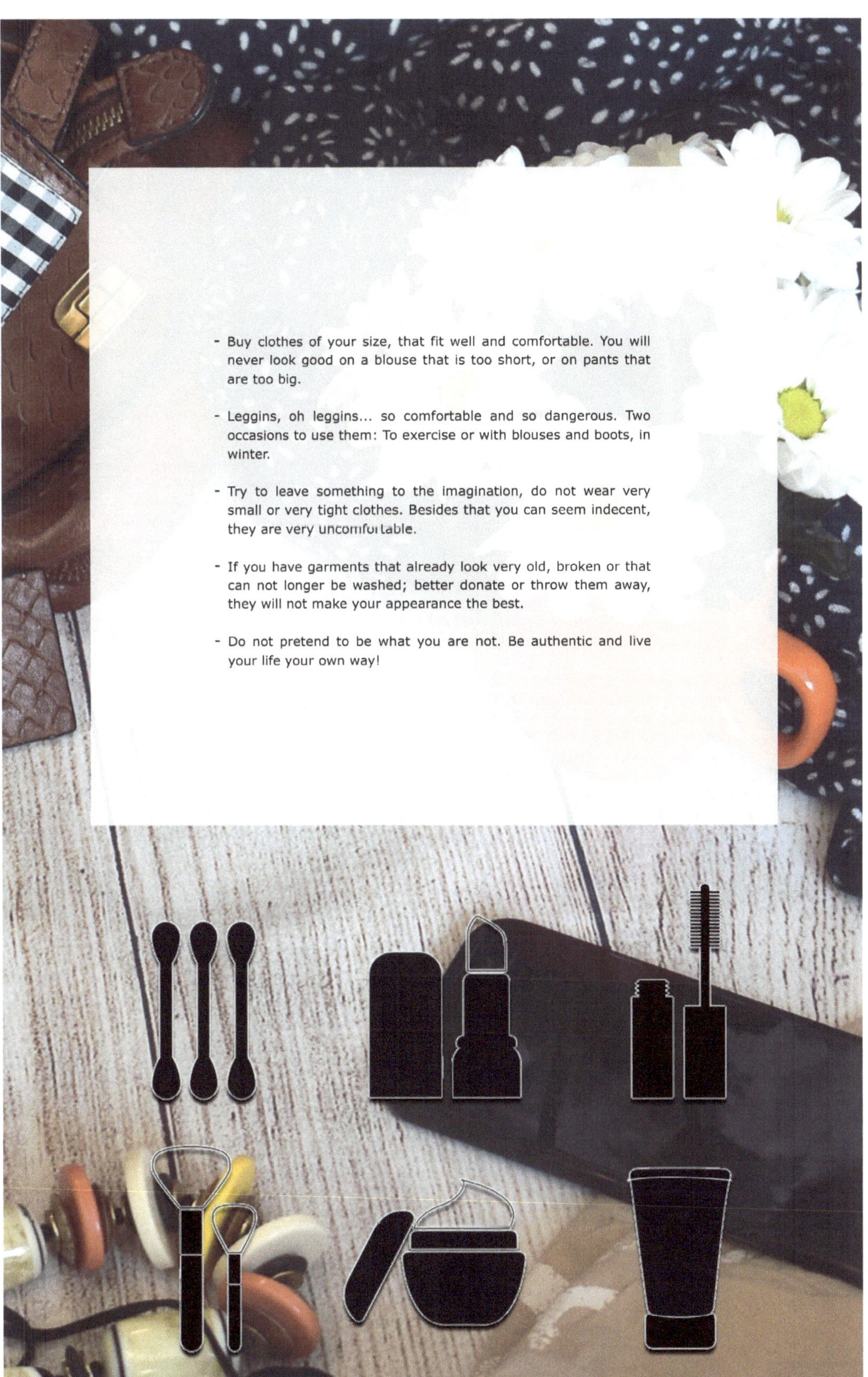

- Buy clothes of your size, that fit well and comfortable. You will never look good on a blouse that is too short, or on pants that are too big.

- Leggins, oh leggins... so comfortable and so dangerous. Two occasions to use them: To exercise or with blouses and boots, in winter.

- Try to leave something to the imagination, do not wear very small or very tight clothes. Besides that you can seem indecent, they are very uncomfortable.

- If you have garments that already look very old, broken or that can not longer be washed; better donate or throw them away, they will not make your appearance the best.

- Do not pretend to be what you are not. Be authentic and live your life your own way!

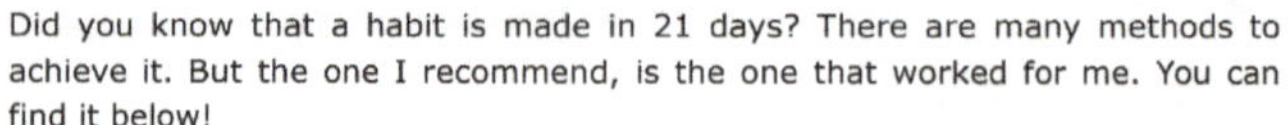

Did you know that a habit is made in 21 days? There are many methods to achieve it. But the one I recommend, is the one that worked for me. You can find it below!

		1	2	3	4	5
6	7	8	9	10	11	12
13	14	15	16	17	18	19
20	21	22	23	24	25	26
27	28	29	30	31		

Take a calendar and write on the 21 days the habit you are proposing. Every day cross it out with your favorite color. At the end it will be easier for you to perform the task you proposed. Do it!

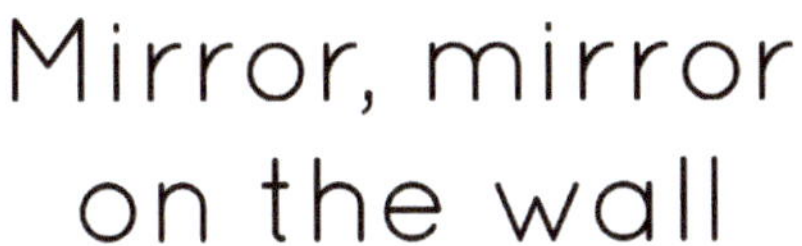

Mirror, mirror on the wall

We already have a very good way traveled. We analyzed our body type, we learned about clothing recommendations, dress codes, etc. Now, it is time to discover our face type, or also called visagism.

It is advisable to know our face type to be able to highlight our positive traits, and minimize the negatives. That is how we will achieve a harmonious face.

There are many types of faces, but to facilitate the process they have been classified into five.

1. **Oval**
2. **Round**
3. **Square**
4. **Heart**
5. **Rectangle**

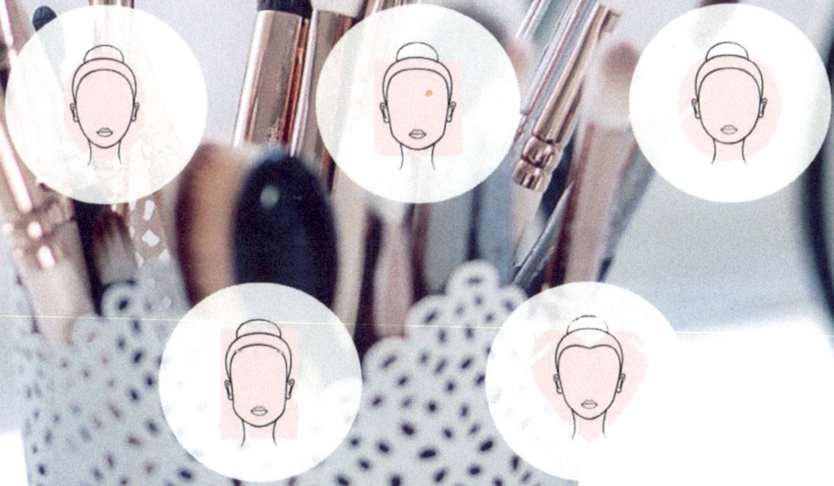

Face type

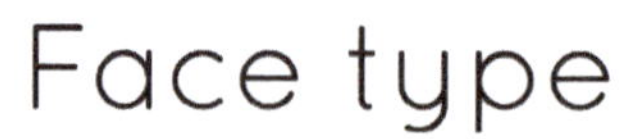

Place the picture of your face here.

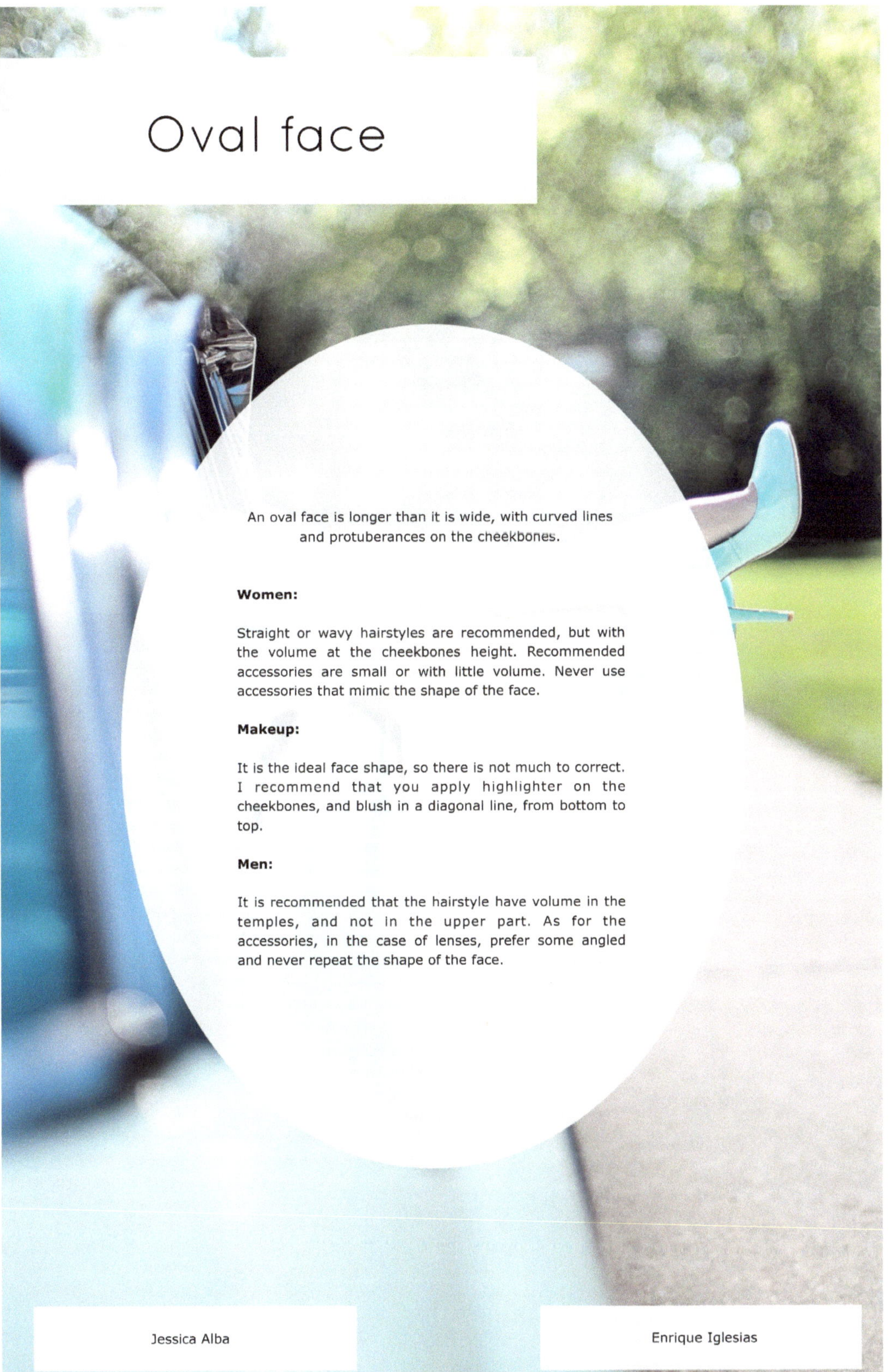

Oval face

An oval face is longer than it is wide, with curved lines and protuberances on the cheekbones.

Women:

Straight or wavy hairstyles are recommended, but with the volume at the cheekbones height. Recommended accessories are small or with little volume. Never use accessories that mimic the shape of the face.

Makeup:

It is the ideal face shape, so there is not much to correct. I recommend that you apply highlighter on the cheekbones, and blush in a diagonal line, from bottom to top.

Men:

It is recommended that the hairstyle have volume in the temples, and not in the upper part. As for the accessories, in the case of lenses, prefer some angled and never repeat the shape of the face.

Jessica Alba

Enrique Iglesias

Round face

A round face has the same length and width, its lines are curved and the cheekbones prominent.

Women:

Prefer straight hairstyle, accessories with angles or spikes. It is not advisable to use volume on the face. If you use necklines, prefer those that are in the form of a triangle and avoid rounded ones.

Makeup:

The shape of the eyebrows will be angular, and the curved shapes must be avoided. Blush should be applied diagonally and from bottom to top. Matte finishes will look better on you, avoid highlighter and lip gloss.

Men:

Hairstyle without much volume on the temples, but in the upper part. Prefer lenses and collars with straight and angled designs.

Kristen Dunst

Zach Galifianakis

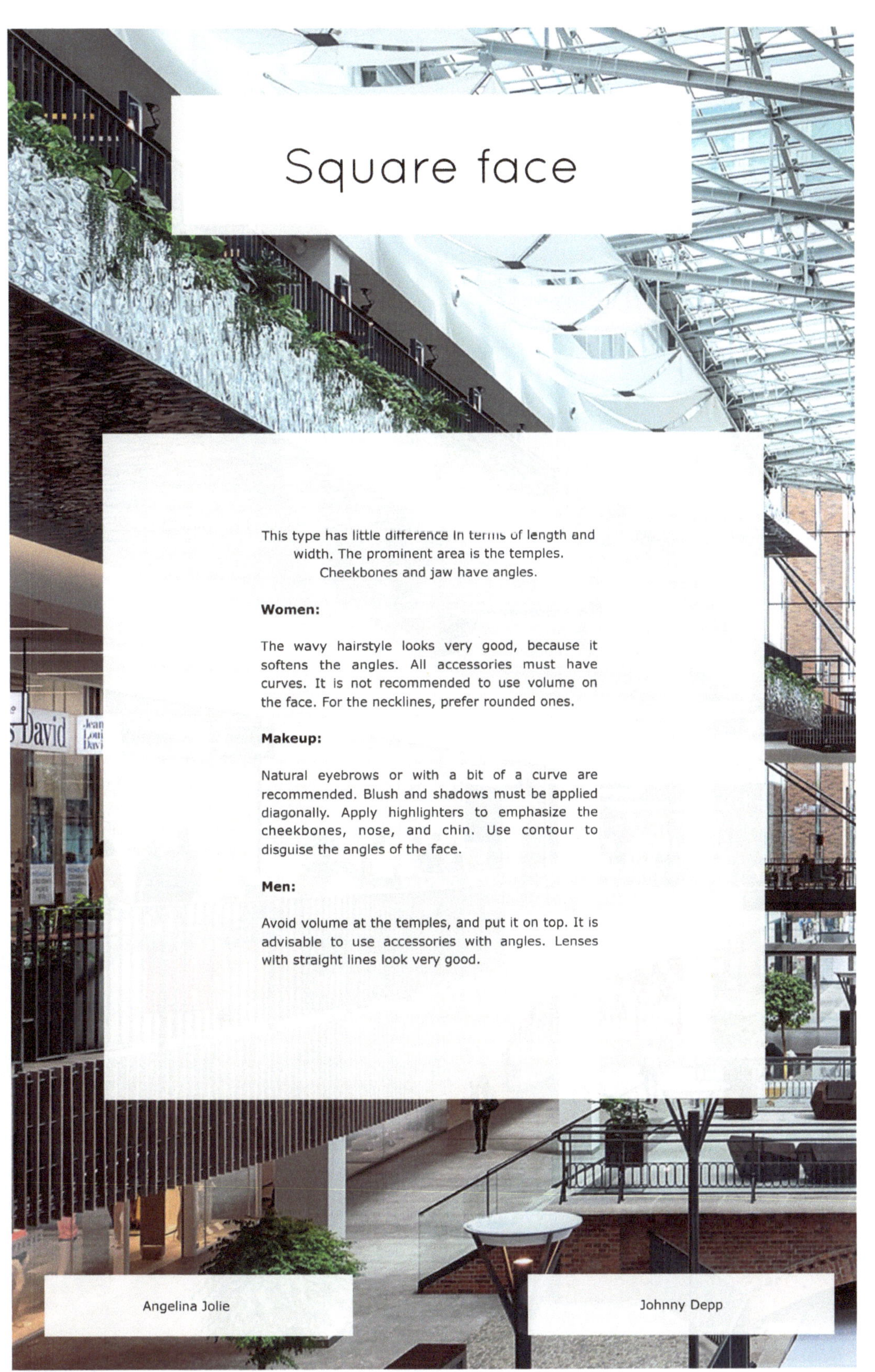

Square face

This type has little difference in terms of length and width. The prominent area is the temples. Cheekbones and jaw have angles.

Women:

The wavy hairstyle looks very good, because it softens the angles. All accessories must have curves. It is not recommended to use volume on the face. For the necklines, prefer rounded ones.

Makeup:

Natural eyebrows or with a bit of a curve are recommended. Blush and shadows must be applied diagonally. Apply highlighters to emphasize the cheekbones, nose, and chin. Use contour to disguise the angles of the face.

Men:

Avoid volume at the temples, and put it on top. It is advisable to use accessories with angles. Lenses with straight lines look very good.

Angelina Jolie

Johnny Depp

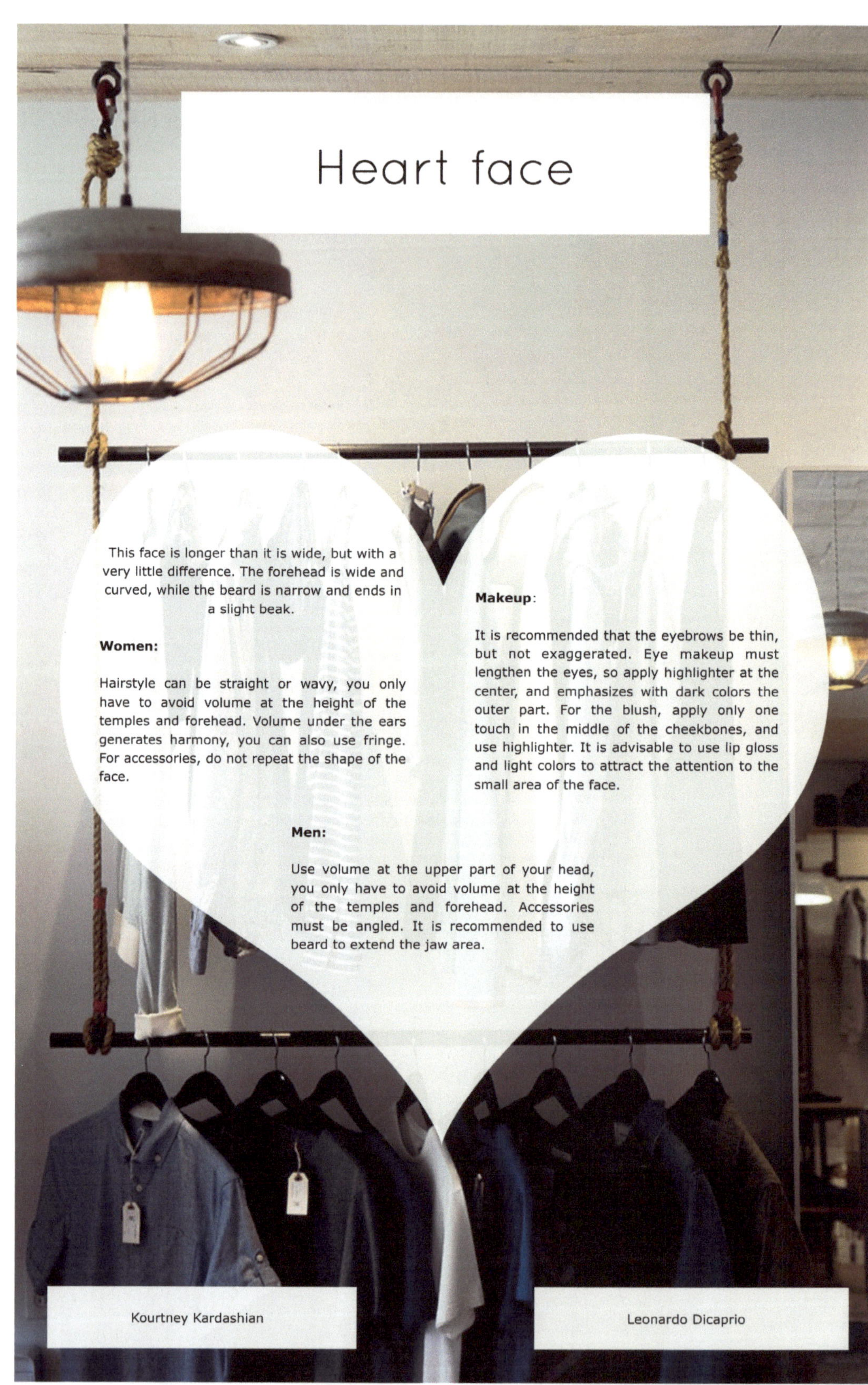

Heart face

This face is longer than it is wide, but with a very little difference. The forehead is wide and curved, while the beard is narrow and ends in a slight beak.

Women:

Hairstyle can be straight or wavy, you only have to avoid volume at the height of the temples and forehead. Volume under the ears generates harmony, you can also use fringe. For accessories, do not repeat the shape of the face.

Men:

Use volume at the upper part of your head, you only have to avoid volume at the height of the temples and forehead. Accessories must be angled. It is recommended to use beard to extend the jaw area.

Makeup:

It is recommended that the eyebrows be thin, but not exaggerated. Eye makeup must lengthen the eyes, so apply highlighter at the center, and emphasizes with dark colors the outer part. For the blush, apply only one touch in the middle of the cheekbones, and use highlighter. It is advisable to use lip gloss and light colors to attract the attention to the small area of the face.

Kourtney Kardashian

Leonardo Dicaprio

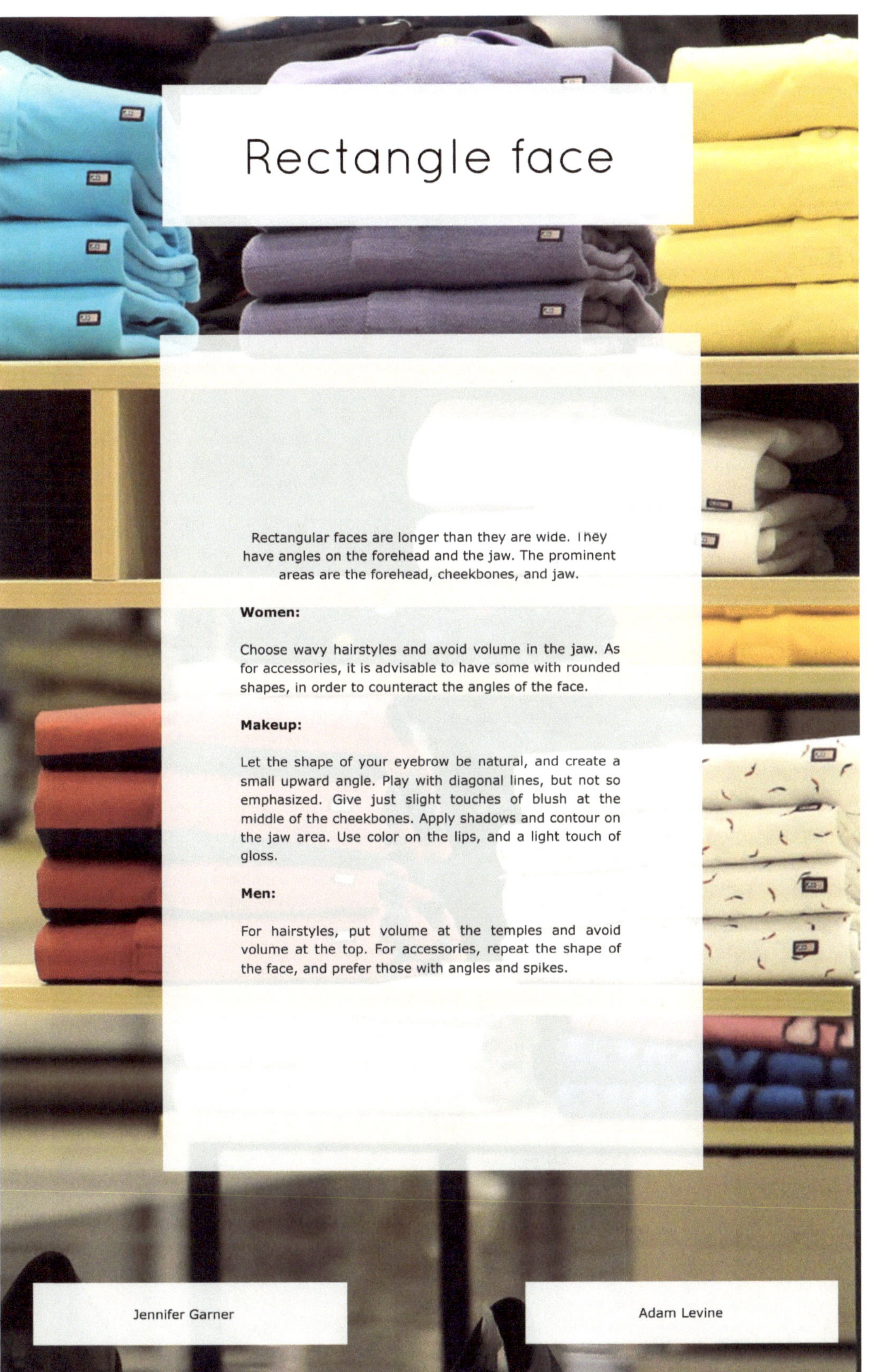

Rectangle face

Rectangular faces are longer than they are wide. They have angles on the forehead and the jaw. The prominent areas are the forehead, cheekbones, and jaw.

Women:

Choose wavy hairstyles and avoid volume in the jaw. As for accessories, it is advisable to have some with rounded shapes, in order to counteract the angles of the face.

Makeup:

Let the shape of your eyebrow be natural, and create a small upward angle. Play with diagonal lines, but not so emphasized. Give just slight touches of blush at the middle of the cheekbones. Apply shadows and contour on the jaw area. Use color on the lips, and a light touch of gloss.

Men:

For hairstyles, put volume at the temples and avoid volume at the top. For accessories, repeat the shape of the face, and prefer those with angles and spikes.

Jennifer Garner

Adam Levine

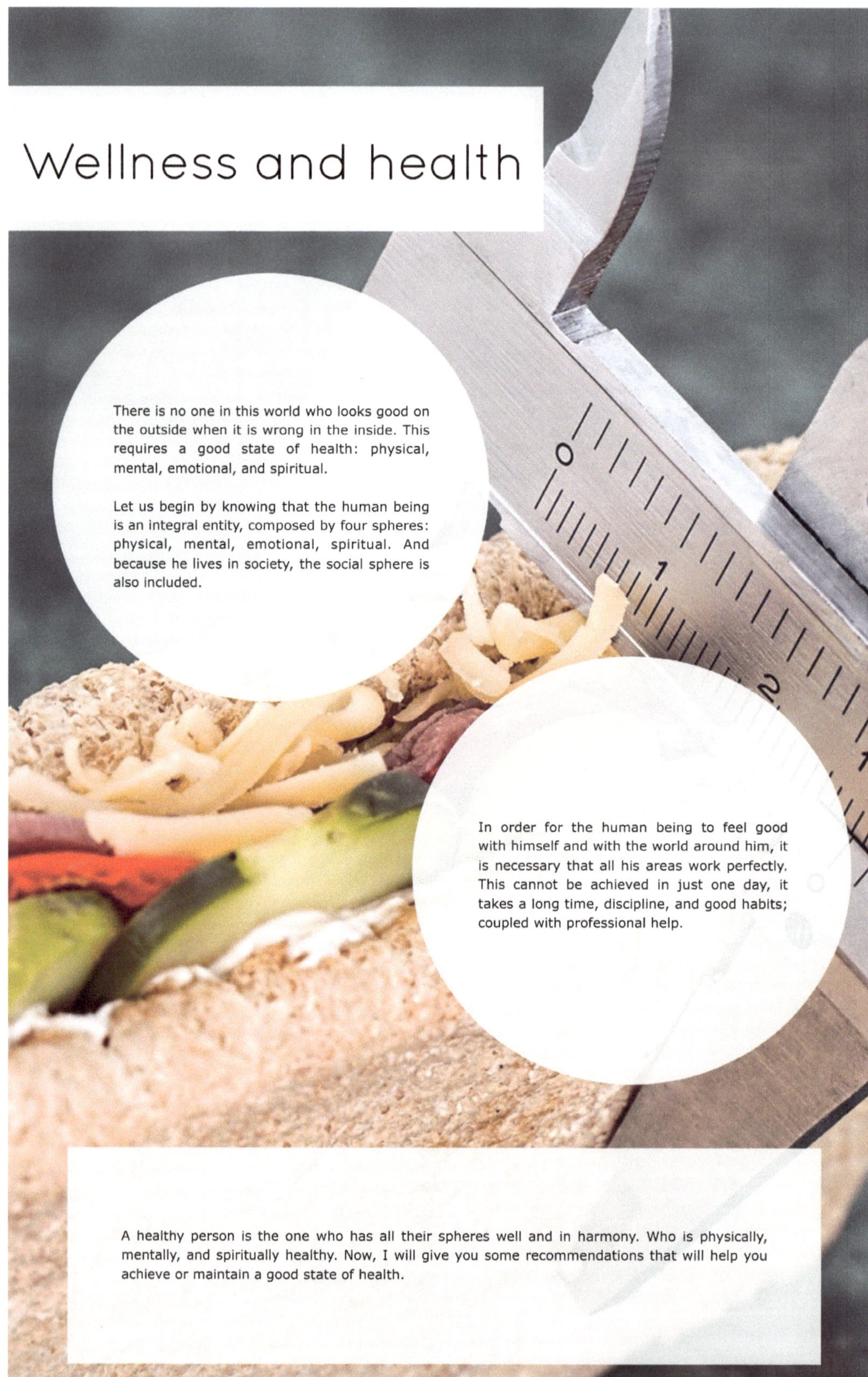

Wellness and health

There is no one in this world who looks good on the outside when it is wrong in the inside. This requires a good state of health: physical, mental, emotional, and spiritual.

Let us begin by knowing that the human being is an integral entity, composed by four spheres: physical, mental, emotional, spiritual. And because he lives in society, the social sphere is also included.

In order for the human being to feel good with himself and with the world around him, it is necessary that all his areas work perfectly. This cannot be achieved in just one day, it takes a long time, discipline, and good habits; coupled with professional help.

A healthy person is the one who has all their spheres well and in harmony. Who is physically, mentally, and spiritually healthy. Now, I will give you some recommendations that will help you achieve or maintain a good state of health.

Health recommendations

To have a healthy diet it is recommended to eat fruits and vegetables, five per day. A way to consume them is as: snack, entrance, dessert, and sweet craving.

It is recommended to include in the diet whole grains, either in: five grains bread, multigrain, rye, flaxseed, corn tortillas, among others.

Your body needs water to be able to function, so it is recommended to take eight glasses of water a day. My tip is always to carry a bottle of water.

Fried, battered, or breaded food should be avoided. Always prefer to grill or oven.

A good recommendation and a very simple one, is to order half portions instead of the whole dish. Except for fruits and vegetables. For example: Two slices of pepperoni cheese pizza have 850 calories, while a single slice has 500 calories. Good advice, right?

To measure the portions of what we eat there are some references:

A. Limit your portions of pasta to half a cup, or the size of your fist closed.
B. Avoid eating red meat, the measure would be 100 grams or the palm of your hand.
C. The tip of your index finger is the portion of butter you should be consuming.
D. The tip of your thumb is the portion of peanut butter you should eat.
E. A cup of ice cream is enough, same as the size of your closed fist.

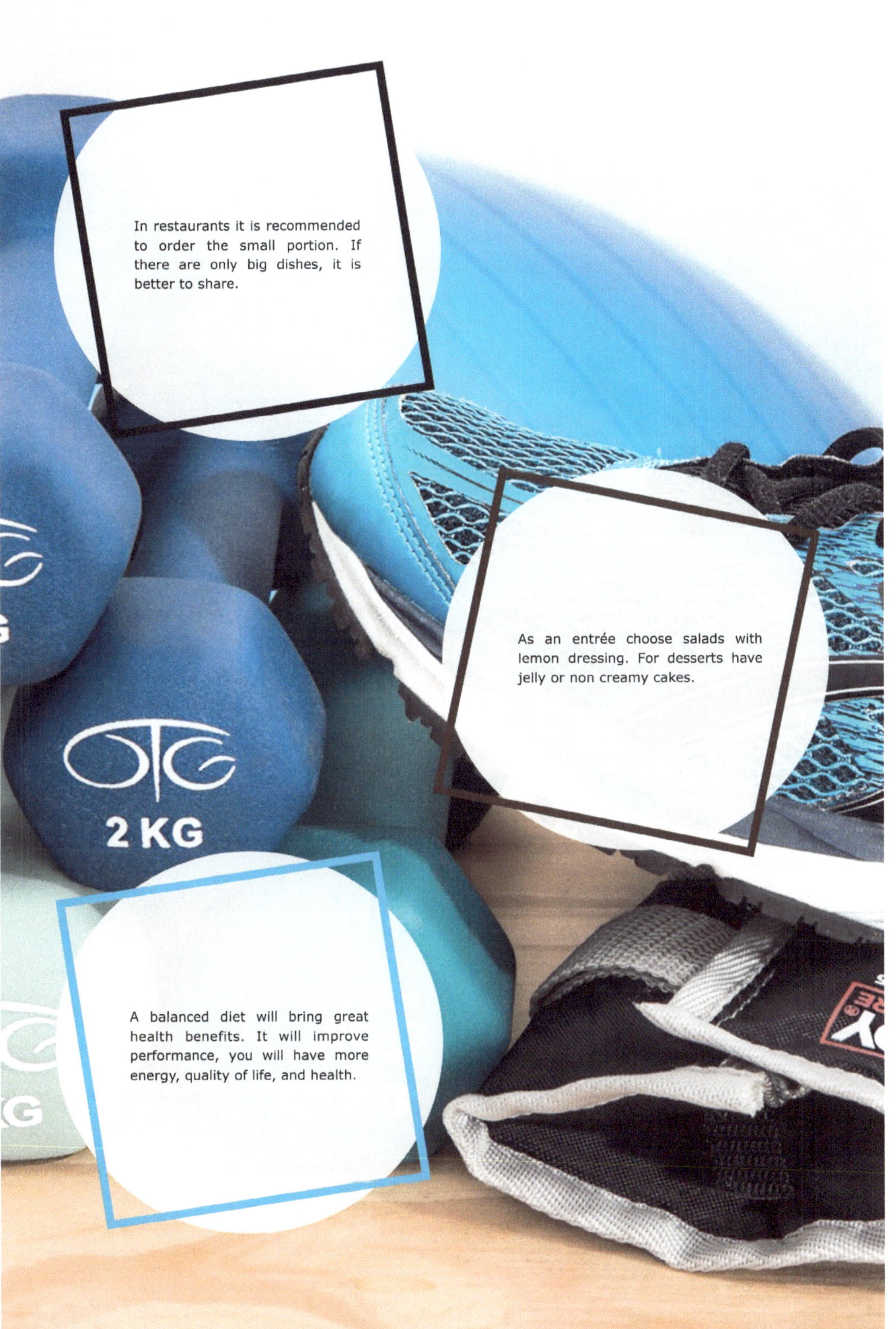
In restaurants it is recommended to order the small portion. If there are only big dishes, it is better to share.
As an entrée choose salads with lemon dressing. For desserts have jelly or non creamy cakes.
A balanced diet will bring great health benefits. It will improve performance, you will have more energy, quality of life, and health.
OTG 2 KG

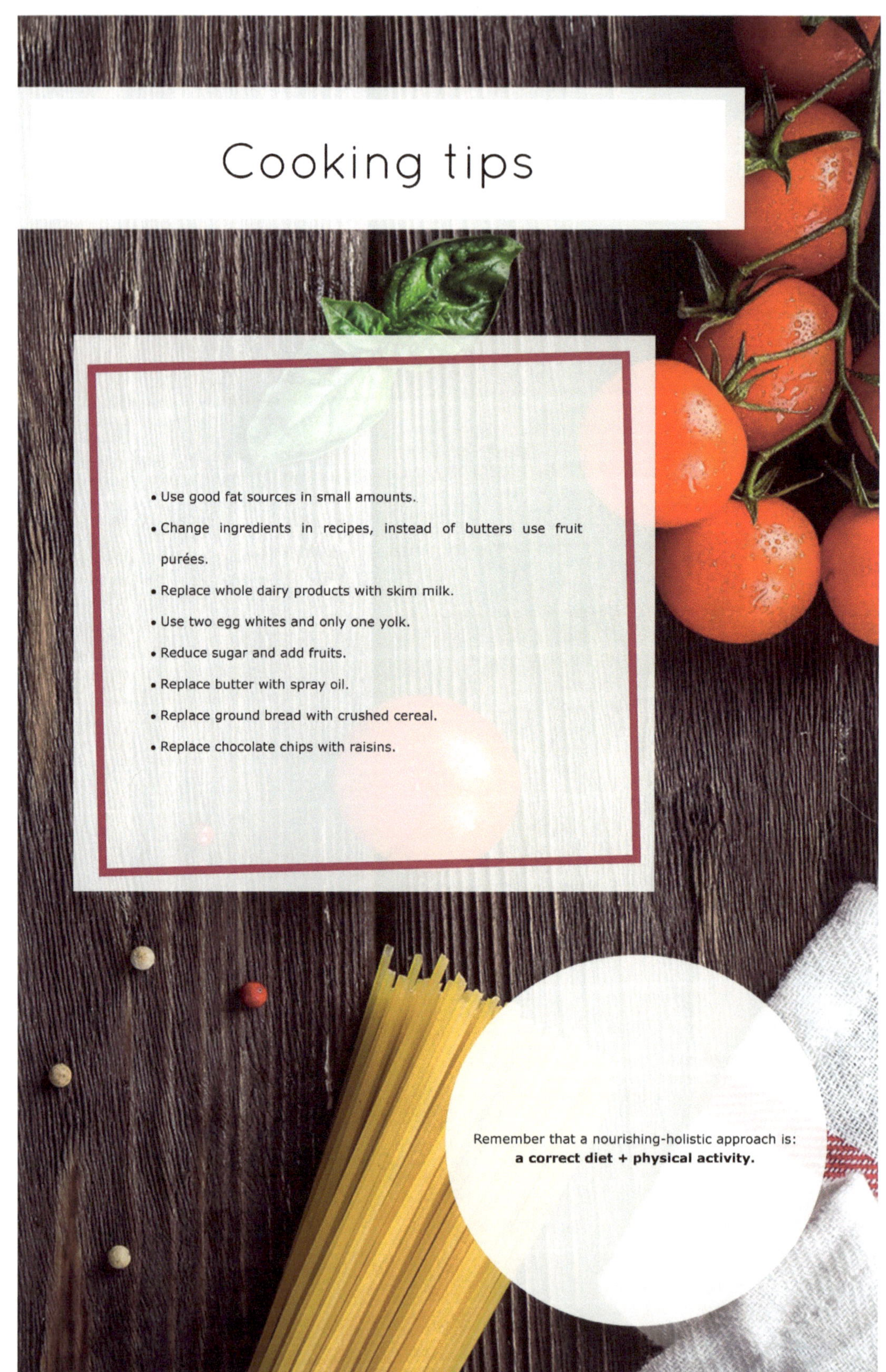

Cooking tips

- Use good fat sources in small amounts.
- Change ingredients in recipes, instead of butters use fruit purées.
- Replace whole dairy products with skim milk.
- Use two egg whites and only one yolk.
- Reduce sugar and add fruits.
- Replace butter with spray oil.
- Replace ground bread with crushed cereal.
- Replace chocolate chips with raisins.

Remember that a nourishing-holistic approach is:
a correct diet + physical activity.

Healthy living habits

Some daily habits that will help you get a healthy lifestyle are:

1 hour of exercise
2 liters of water
3 cups of tea
4 servings of fruits
5 meals
6 songs that inspire you
7 minutes of laughter
8 hours sleep
9 pages of a book
10 minutes of meditation

This habits will make your life happier and healthier, follow them and create the best version of yourself.

Do it for yourself!

Notes

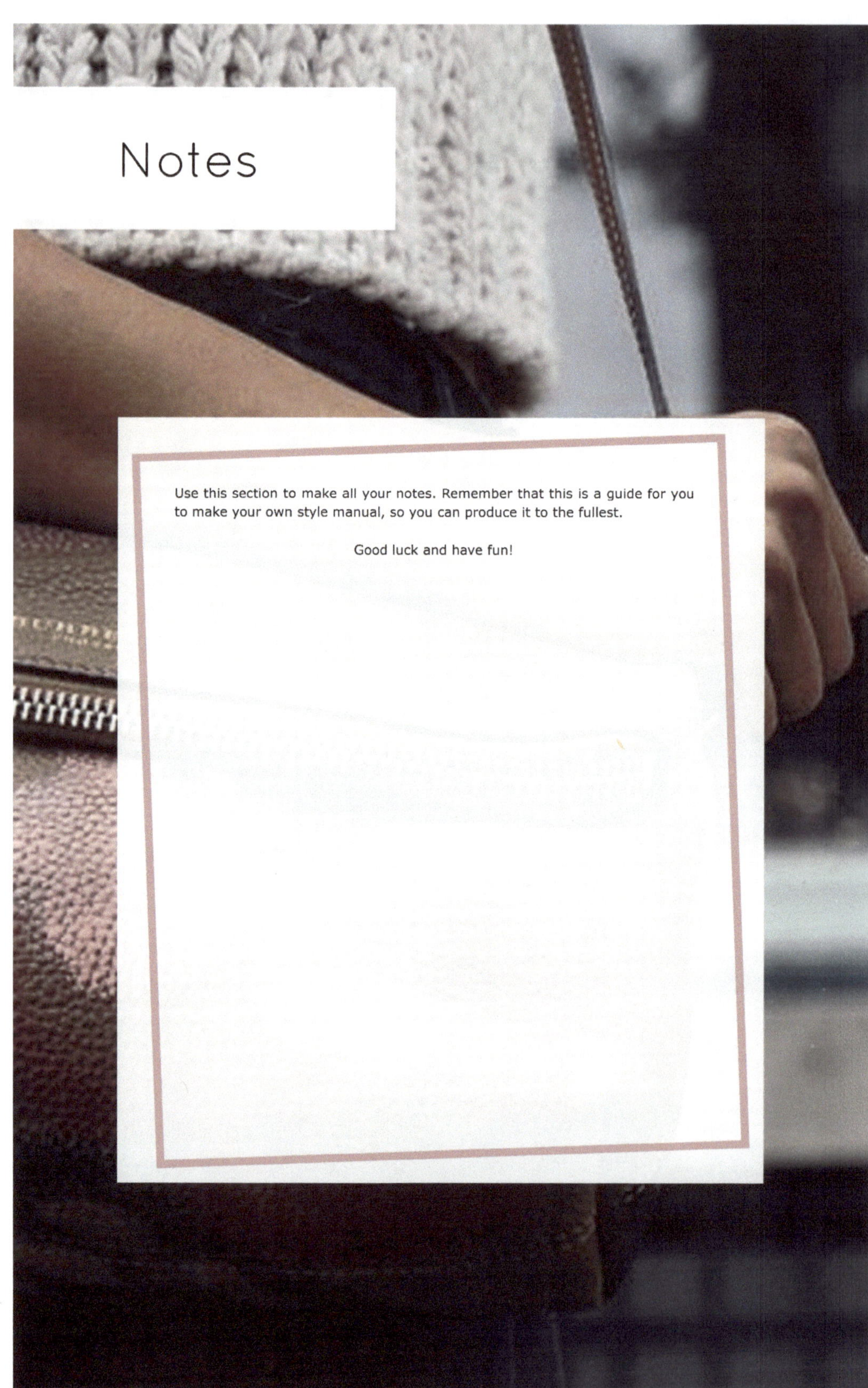

Use this section to make all your notes. Remember that this is a guide for you to make your own style manual, so you can produce it to the fullest.

Good luck and have fun!

Notes

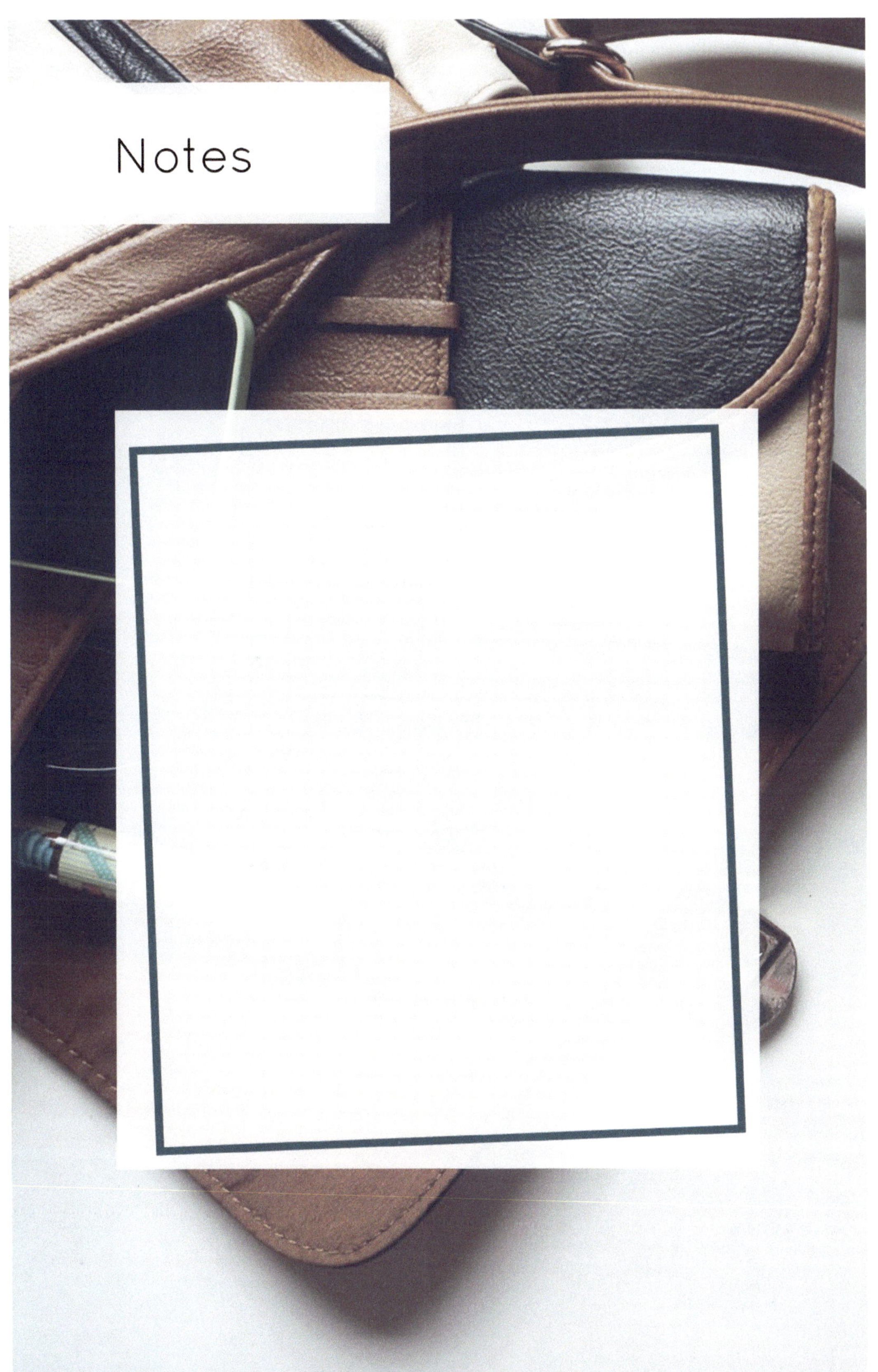

Notes

Notes

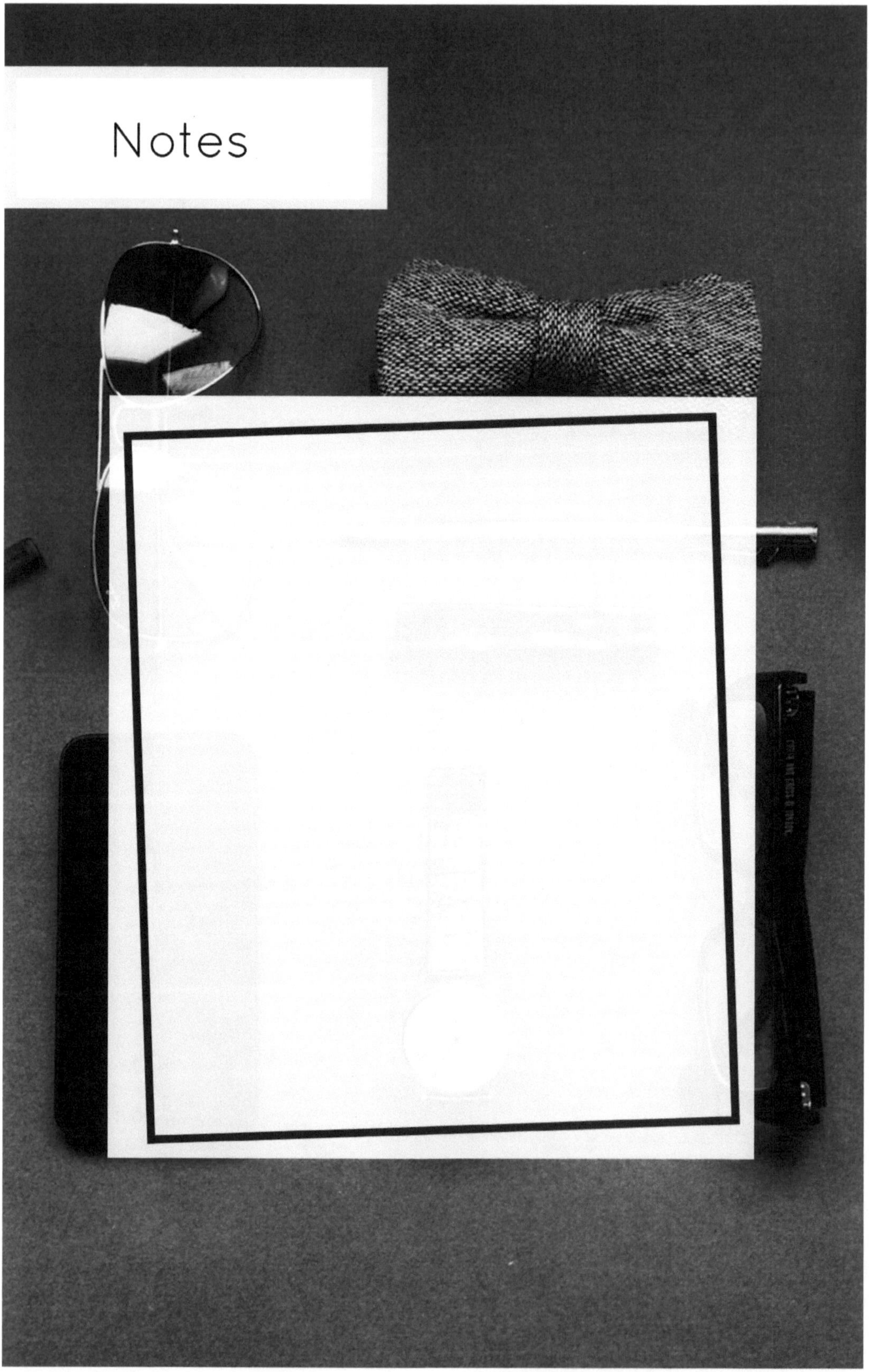

Notes
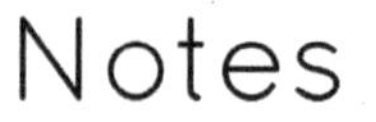

You have reached the end of the manual, and let me congratulate you because now you know how to make a better version of yourself. Not just to look good, but to make you feel great about yourself. That is the most important thing.

Let me tell you after all these tips, that beauty is inside the person. It is much prettier an authentic person who loves himself, than one that is empty in the inside, but meets the commercial standards of what is considered "beautiful."

Do not get carried away by the stereotypes of the fashion industry, almost no one meets those parameters. Use the tools and advice I gave you, to highlight your own beauty. If you look good, you will feel good, and vice versa.

Believe me, it is worth waking up a few minutes before, to look perfect the rest of the day. Results will be shown very quickly. People around you will start to tell how good you look. The person you like will look at you. You can even achieve your dream job.

Go ahead and put into practice what you just learned. From now on you are a new person.

I wish you much success!

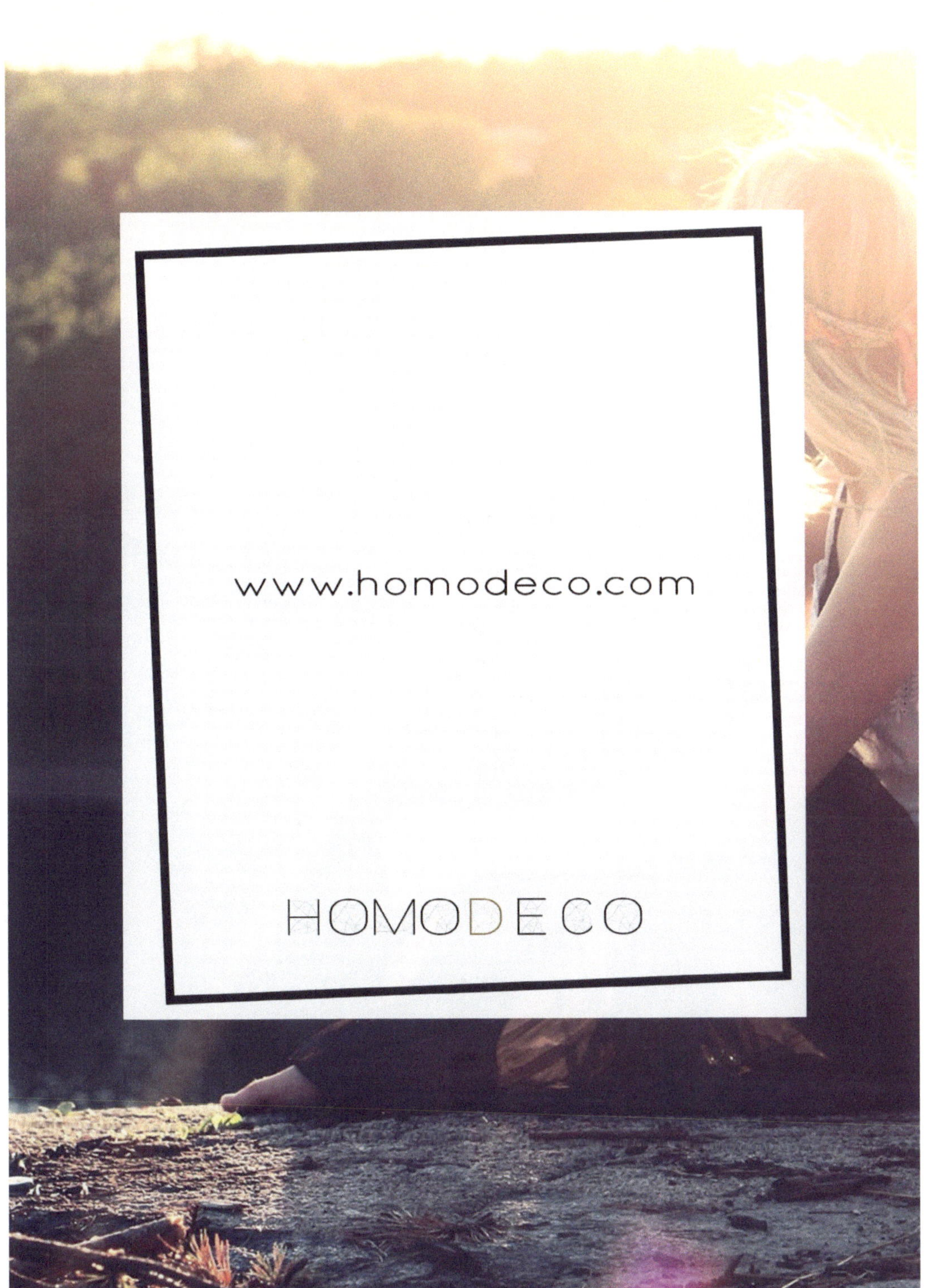

www.homodeco.com
HOMODECO

Feel good, live good!

Do you know how expensive it is to have a Personal Image Consultant? Do not worry about it! Here you have the manual that Image Consultants use to make our clients get the best version of themselves.

In your hands you have endless recommendations and tools that will simplify your life when deciding how to produce yourself for that special moment, or perhaps to go to work, or for whatever you want to.

It does not matter if you are a man, woman, girl, public figure, teenager, entrepreneur, artist, etc. I assure you that what you are about to read will serve as a guide for the rest of your life.

And remember... Your image is worth a thousand words!

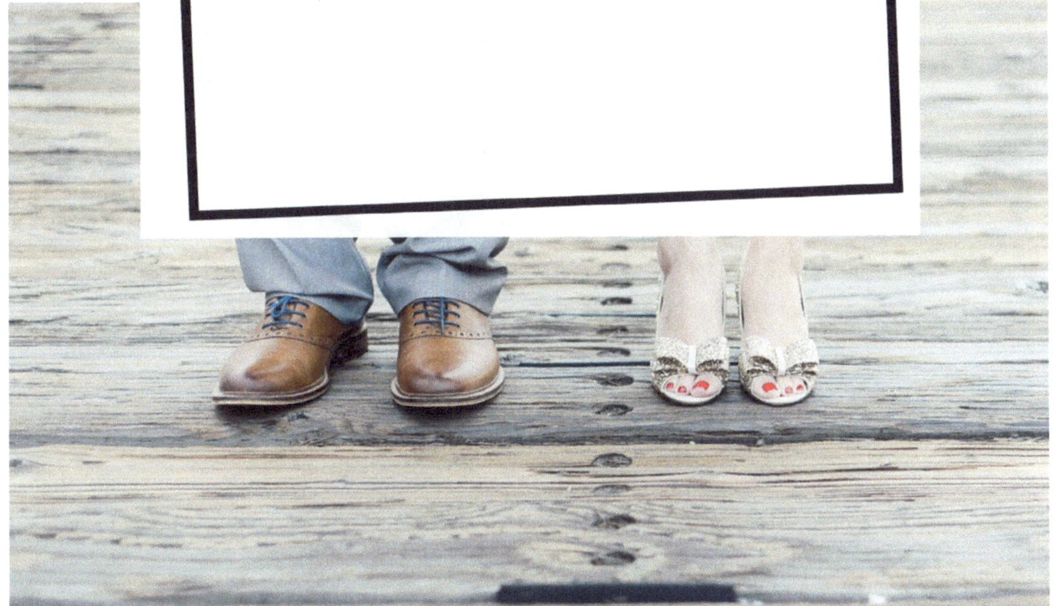